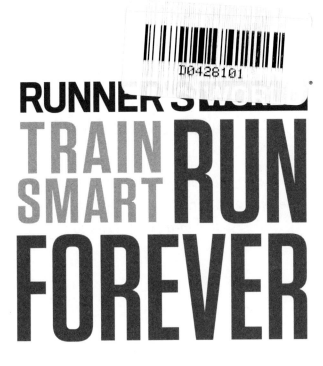

RUNNER'S WORLD
TRAIN SMART RUN
FOREVER

Also by Bill Pierce and Scott Murr:

Runner's World Run Less, Run Faster:
Become a Faster, Stronger Runner with the Revolutionary
3-Run-a-Week Training Program

RUNNER'S WORLD

TRAIN SMART RUN FOREVER

HOW TO BE A FIT AND HEALTHY LIFELONG RUNNER FOLLOWING THE INNOVATIVE 7-HOUR WORKOUT WEEK

From the Experts at *FIRST*®

BILL PIERCE
and SCOTT MURR

RODALE.

RODALE wellness

Live happy. Be healthy. Get inspired.

Sign up today to get exclusive access to our authors, exclusive bonuses, and the most authoritative, useful, and cutting-edge information on health, wellness, fitness, and living your life to the fullest.

Visit us online at RodaleWellness.com

Join us at RodaleWellness.com/Join

Rodale books may be purchased for business or promotional use or for special sales. For information, please write to:
Special Markets Department, Rodale, Inc., 733 Third Avenue, New York, NY 10017

Runner's World is a registered trademark of Rodale Inc.

Printed in the United States of America

Rodale Inc. makes every effort to use acid-free ♾, recycled paper ♻.

Book design by Joanna Williams

Photographs: page 42: Thomas Alder; pages vi, 144, 190, 250: Olivier Blanchard; pages 173–217: Jeremy Fleming; pages xxviii, 218: Marathon Foto; page viii: Santiago Morel; pages xii, 24, 68, 106, 132, 146, 155, 170, 238: Scott Murr

Library of Congress Cataloging-in-Publication Data is on file with the Publisher.

ISBN-13: 978-1-62336-746-6 paperback

Distributed to the trade by Macmillan

2 4 6 8 10 9 7 5 3 1 paperback

RODALE.

Follow us @RodaleBooks on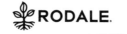

We inspire health, healing, happiness, and love in the world.
Starting with you.

To the thousands of runners around the globe who have shared with us their FIRST training program experiences

and

to all who are pursuing a lifetime of running.

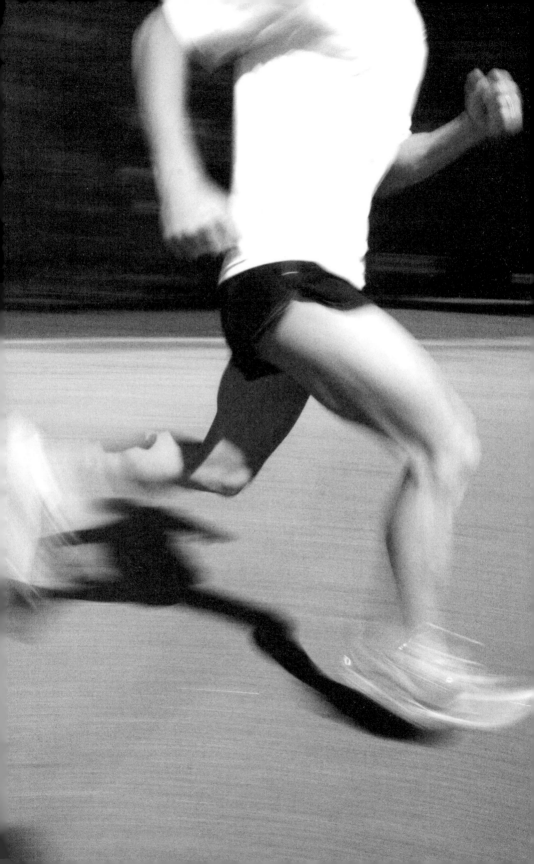

CONTENTS

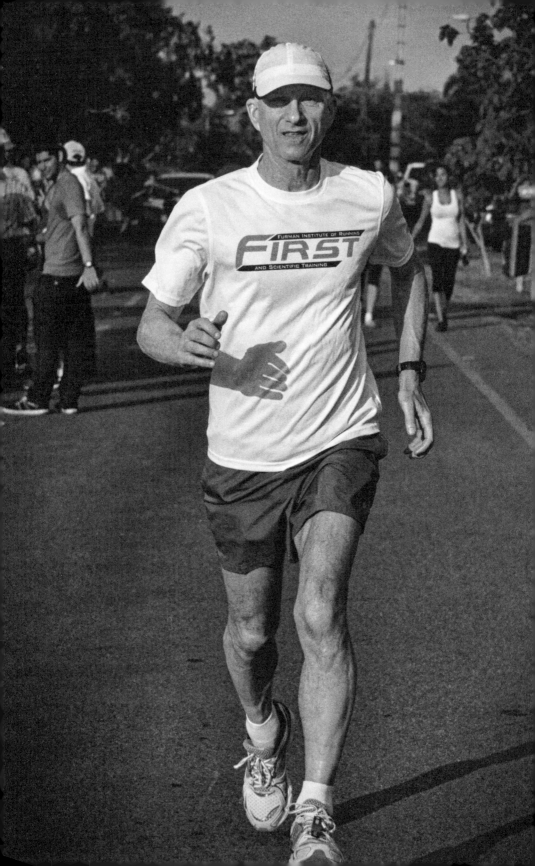

FOREWORD

WHEN YOU FIRST MEET HIM, in his crisp button-down shirts and pressed khaki pants, with his tea drinker's manners and opera devotee's charm, Bill Pierce comes across as the college professor and university administrator he is.

What you may not immediately apprehend is that this man is fierce. His trim waistline hasn't inched up since his days of basket-ball stardom on high school courts in West Virginia and on three Southern Conference teams at Davidson College. Beneath that Bruce Wayne exterior is a 60-something superhero—an athlete committed to performing puke-inducing workouts, a butt-kicking competitor. Just being with Bill makes you want to stand up straighter, swear off Cheez-Its, and get your lazy self to the track. It's never anything he says. Always polite and courteous, Bill doesn't offer unsolicited advice. But when you ask for his help, he gives.

When Bill invited me to come to Furman University to talk to his first-year students who had read my book on running, I said yes. During my visit, when he proposed to measure my body fat, hector me to reach my lactate threshold, and stand beside the treadmill as I maxed out my VO_2, I said *no freaking way*. I was, I thought, beyond caring about my marathon times. My PRs were long behind me.

But spend enough time with him and you will fall under Bill's spell. You begin to wonder if maybe you could get faster. You resolve to push yourself harder. You want, most of all, not to disappoint him.

Like many humans, I regularly lie to myself about lots of things, including my level of fitness. If I compare myself to most people, I'm doing okay. But I've never wanted "most people" to be my control group; I prefer to keep company with those who are excellent. For much of my running life, I've done my long runs with younger men. These days, when I tell myself it's fine that I can't keep up—they're younger! they're men!—I'm lying. It doesn't feel fine. It sucks.

So after I'd met with the Furman students, I submitted and let Bill's team perform a battery of expensive tests on me. I whined the whole time and then quailed at the results. The data showed I was not as fit as I wanted to believe. Data, scientists like to remind us, don't lie. And data don't give a hoot about our feelings.

Hoots were, however, given by Bill. As he consoled me, he talked about the inevitable downward slither we can expect as we age and reminded me that if you want to run fast, you have to run fast. Bill invited me to come back for one of his FIRST retreats. This time, I said *yes, please.*

At the retreat, I met a group of people as culturally diverse as they were serious about running. We sat in classrooms listening to engaging lectures and lay relaxed on the bed of the DEXA machine—until we discovered that while we may have looked trim and fit, many of us were padded with pace-slowing fat. We ran on treadmills wearing Darth Vader masks, stopping every few minutes to let otherwise pleasant people stick needles in our fingers. As often happens when folks suffer together, we bonded.

Since I'd spent years writing for magazines about running, I knew much of what we were taught. However, I'd managed to ignore almost everything and implement none of it into my training, which had, by then, deteriorated to the ignoble level of a recreational jogger.

The FIRST retreat made me determined to get faster. Following orders has never been my strong suit, but when Bill agreed to coach me, I found myself thrilled never to have to think about my running. I just did whatever Bill told me to do. The tables in *Runner's World Run Less, Run Faster* gave me exact workouts at precise paces. While I occasionally went on unsanctioned dog runs (I had a puppy) and couldn't resist entering beloved races that were not in my best (training) interest, the satisfaction of completing each tempo run or track workout, and then being able to report to Bill and bask in his approval, made the experience a joy.

And at the age of 50, I ran my fastest marathon in 7 years.

If you believe that you are immune to the ravages of age, well, good luck to you. I hope Santa or the Easter Bunny brings you eternal youth. But if you want to keep running into your dotage and you're open to receiving help and advice to be able to keep doing what you love, this book is for you.

Here, Bill Pierce and his equally hardcore coauthor, Scott Murr—father to two teenagers and six-time finisher of the Ironman Triathlon World Championships in Kona, Hawaii—tell you what you need to know. Ignore their wisdom at your peril.

Rachel Toor
Professor of Creative Writing
Eastern Washington University

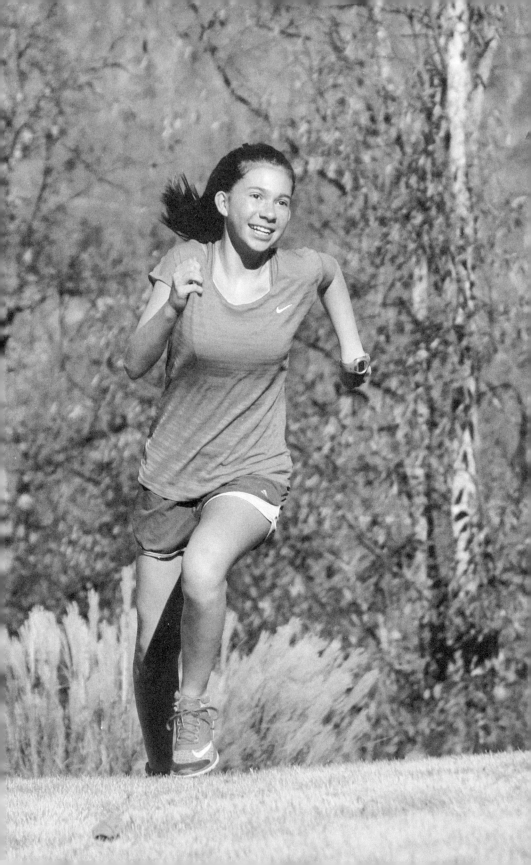

PREFACE

IN 1983, I ACCEPTED A position as assistant professor of health and physical education at Furman University in Greenville, South Carolina. As a distance runner, I welcomed the move from beautiful but cold and snowy Idaho to the sunny South. Even with its hot, humid summers, Greenville, located in the Upstate of South Carolina near the foothills of the Blue Ridge Mountains, offers a climate conducive to year-round training and an active running community. I was attracted to Furman because of its emphasis on a required fitness-concepts course for all students. As the department chair since 1984, I have led the institution's commitment to promote wellness among the students, faculty, and staff. I am gratified by the many members of the campus community who have come to enjoy running, cycling, swimming, and a broad array of fitness activities.

Two members of the Furman community significantly influenced my personal life and professional career. Scott Murr was a senior health and physical education major when I arrived at Furman. He was an outstanding student and a fitness enthusiast. We soon began running and racing together. For 3½ decades we have shared those activities and mutual interests. Three years after I began my teaching at Furman, I hired exercise physiologist Ray Moss. Ray had been teaching at a medical school in Texas and brought a wealth of knowledge and skill to Furman. Almost immediately after arriving at Furman, Ray designed, built, and developed a first-class human-performance laboratory with the fitness-assessment capabilities needed for testing runners' physiological parameters.

Scott, who joined our faculty after he earned a doctorate in exercise science, Ray, and I spent thousands of hours discussing fitness and training methods over the next 15 years before the three of us founded the Furman Institute of Running and Scientific Training (FIRST).

We established FIRST with an aim of assisting local runners with their training and racing. We launched FIRST by offering four lectures per month free to the public on various aspects of running. Then followed a commitment to volunteer our time as a public service to promote smart training based on our personal experiences and our expertise as exercise scientists. The well-attended lectures brought requests for training programs.

We began sharing our own training schedules with the runners. As the lecture presentations and training schedules for various race distances piled up, I started trying to organize them into a coherent training manual.

It was about that time that Amby Burfoot, then the executive editor of *Runner's World*, saw our Web site and contacted me to find out what we were doing. After I described the research studies that we were conducting and our effort to promote running in the community, he said that he would like to visit our campus and learn more about FIRST.

Amby's visit was a joy. We talked running nonstop for 4 days along with doing workouts together. Any time spent with Amby Burfoot results in a running education. No one in the past 50 years has observed more running competitions, interacted with more world-class runners, interviewed more experts on running, and written more about every aspect of running than Amby Burfoot. He was intrigued with what we were attempting to do because we were not engaging in a for-profit venture. We still aren't. That is what has made it fun, interesting, and enjoyable for us.

Scott, Ray, and I were confident that our training program based on three weekly run workouts coupled with two aerobic cross-training workouts was effective. However, we decided that before we could tout that program to the public, we needed to test it with a wide range of runners. We spent 3 years conducting three 16-week training programs with female and male runners with ages ranging from twenties to sixties. They were all tested in the human-performance laboratory before and after the training programs. The positive improvement experienced by the runners after following our prescribed regimens gave us proof that even veteran runners could improve by adhering to our program's specific workouts tailored to their fitness level.

Amby Burfoot interviewed the runners from these research studies. What happened next changed FIRST and our lives like no other event in our professional careers. Amby wrote a six-page feature article in the August 2005 issue of *Runner's World*. Never doubt the power of the press. From the day that issue hit the newsstands, we have been contacted continuously by runners from around the world. That is because the article appeared in the European, southern Africa, and Australia/New Zealand editions of *Runner's World*, as well as its being posted on the *Runner's World's* Web site. Some folks e-mail us, some call, and others come to Greenville to visit us.

Amby also encouraged us to write a book. I explained that I thought a training manual that I was developing would be adequate, but he insisted it should be a book.

Not long after Amby's insistence on a book, I was interviewed by Tara Parker-Pope, who was then writing for the *Wall Street Journal,* for an article about half-marathons. Hours after the article was published, I was contacted by a New York book agent, Barrett Neville, asking if I was interested in writing a book. After conversations with him over the next 2 weeks, we began preparing a proposal. We accepted an offer from Rodale, publisher of *Runner's World,* and a year later *Runner's World Run Less, Run Faster* was published. Five years later, we updated the book with a second edition. Because the book and the concept have been embraced by so many, we continue to enjoy a widespread relationship with runners.

The book gave us the opportunity to interact with runners from around the world. Whether it is elderly women in India racing in colorful saris or runners equipped with high-tech GPS watches, iPods, compression socks and sleeves, and the latest trendy shoes, runners come in all shapes, sizes, and ages around the globe. I keep trying to understand the reasons behind this soaring popularity.

I have been running for more than 50 years, going back to junior high school track. It has always been fun for me. Whether it was running to see how fast I could get to my grandmother's house across town, trying to keep up with my big brother racing through the hills of our southern West Virginia home, competing on my college's cinder track, or racing on the roads for the past 40 years, I have always sought and enjoyed the opportunity to run.

The majority of my more than 50,000 miles of training runs has been with Scott, my brother, Don, or both of them. The three of us have enjoyed miles and miles together. Don is 3 years older and Scott is 12 years younger than I am. When the three of us were in our twenties, thirties, and forties, we were highly competitive with one another, never knowing who might win a race or even one of our training runs. As I said, we were very competitive. Training runs were fun because you never knew when someone would break away and the chase would begin.

We have continued to train together—but not necessarily side by side, as we used to do. Don and I can no longer keep up with Scott. We run on the track at the same time but stick to our own pace. We often add a time handicap to our tempo runs. Scott gives Don and me a few minutes' head start so that we will all finish at nearly the same time. That keeps a competitive element in our playful running. For our long runs, we impose a distance handicap on the younger Scott. Don and I may run 15 miles while Scott runs 17 miles, which will have us finish the last mile or so together.

The fact is, all three of us have had long running careers and wish to continue our regular training and occasional racing. At the time of publication, I am 67, Don is 70, and Scott is 55. Even sprightly Scott has begun to experience the effects of age on his training and racing. Our conversations today often include thoughts about what we must do to be able to enjoy running into our old age. We want to use our experience, observations, and knowledge to craft a plan that will reduce the likelihood of our having to stop running as so many of our peers have had to do. We remind one another to be smart about our training.

I have run 42 marathons over the past 38 years. Don and I have seen our consistent sub-2:50 times creep gradually to 3:10 to 3:30 to 3:45 until we exceeded 4 hours in the fall of 2015 at the ages of 65 and 68. We have discovered that we are no longer racing the marathon, we are enduring it. Our 20-mile-long training runs were nearly 3 hours in our most recent marathon preparation versus the slightly more than 2 hours of yesteryear. These are significant changes in our training and racing dynamics.

The changes that we have experienced, along with our observations and discussions with many aging runners, led us to rethink smart training. We wish to share with runners age 40 and over how to be smart about their training and to avoid the unhealthy behaviors that many runners adopt as a way to deal with the effects of aging.

One of my favorite aspects of *Runner's World Run Less, Run Faster* is that I could guarantee runners that following the program in most cases would improve their fitness and lead to faster times. We realize that we cannot offer you a guarantee that you can run forever by following the plan featured in this book. However, we believe the plan increases the likelihood of your enjoying running for a lifetime.

Just as I did in *Runner's World Run Less, Run Faster,* I will represent my coauthor, Scott Murr, as the voice of the book.

Bill Pierce
April 2017

INTRODUCTION

EACH TUESDAY AT NOON, MY heart rate soars to its peak, currently 174—30 beats per minute fewer than in 1972—while I try to stand straight, catch my breath, and manipulate the function keys of my running watch to check the time of my last track repeat. This familiar weekly ritual has endured the passage of 4 decades. What has changed? Not much, really. Yes, the numbers on the watch face have grown considerably, but the feeling generated from the effort is the same. If I did not have that watch, maybe I would not know the difference. But the younger, faster runners who are a lap ahead provide a dose of reality. As we all cool down together, however, our mutual feelings of satisfaction are all the same. Faster times have no ownership of enhanced moods and emotions. That is why running, unlike most other sports, can be enjoyed into old age, but only if you are smart about it.

My colleague, Scott Murr, and I set three goals for this book: (1) to provide information on running and aging, (2) to give training advice, and (3) most importantly, to set out a detailed plan that will enable runners in their forties and older to continue running for—well, forever.

We, like most runners, have made mistakes misguided by our

exuberance with each improvement in our impatience to become faster. As runners who have experienced and observed the effects of aging, we hope to help you avoid some of those mistakes that can have demoralizing effects on your running or inability to run.

Some information, recommendations, and advice that we offer may be scoffed at by those who have escaped incapacitating interruptions of their running careers. I am reminded of Aleksandr Solzhenitsyn's question in his book about a Stalinist concentration camp, *One Day in the Life of Ivan Denisovich:* "How can you expect a man who is warm to understand a man who is cold?" I suppose that may be true of this book for the uninjured runners who have not begun to slow or experience other irksome aging effects. However, I would advise all runners to hang on to the book, because aging is universal and inevitable.

Since the founding of FIRST (Furman Institute of Running and Scientific Training) in 2003, we have received and responded to more than 10,000 messages from runners. In his popular book *Outliers*, Malcolm Gladwell posited that anyone can master a skill with 10,000 hours of practice. Even if you do not master a skill, there is much that can be learned from doing anything 10,000 times, including reading and replying to messages. Although sometimes we are pressed to do so, we have replied to all the messages.

The questions, statements, and reported performances shared by runners in those messages have influenced our ideas about training and, in particular, how runners can be healthy and fit while pursuing faster race times. Whether we are responding to runners in North America, South America, Europe, Asia, or Australia and New Zealand, the challenges and problems runners report are quite similar. The issues reported by runners have shaped the structure of this book.

The sources for the feedback received from runners are not limited to electronic messages. We have spoken at many events and clinics over the past decade. There is always time after these events to talk with the audience and answer personal questions. Each of these interactions enables us to gain more insight into runners and their issues.

In particular, we have benefited from our relationships with the runners who attended one of our Furman Institute of Running and Scientific Training's Adult Learning and Running Retreats. After spending about 14 hours per day for 4 days with runners, we get to know them quite well. In Chapter 1, we describe what we have learned about runners from these retreats.

We know that not all runners are in a position or inclined to attend a FIRST retreat or one of the other specialized running clinics. We trust that this book will enable us to share a great deal of what you would learn at the retreat. Much of what we know about runners has come from the personalized interactions with the retreat participants.

Many who have attended one of these retreats over the past 10 years have maintained a long-term relationship with us through correspondence or return visits to the Furman campus. We have profiled a number of these runners in this book as examples of the challenges runners encounter.

If you want to develop habits and a training regimen that will allow you to continue running when your peers are shuffling along or spending their days parked in front of a TV, you need to understand how the aging process affects running. In Chapter 2, we present research that describes the aging process. Understanding the physiology of aging can help us develop mental and physical coping strategies to modify our training and expectations.

In Chapter 3, we offer reasons for the soaring popularity of the marathon. We understand why runners are attracted to what is a challenging and satisfying goal; the marathon mystique is a fascinating social phenomenon that is spanning the globe. We don't think that running a marathon is ill-advised. However, we also don't think that it is the healthiest race distance for most runners, especially those of us who are into their sixth or seventh decade. We see many runners base all of their training and racing solely on the marathon. That often leads to injuries, disappointments, poor running form, and chronic fatigue.

Should you be concerned about whether years of dedicated endurance training can have ill effects on your cardiovascular health? Numerous large studies have shown that the benefits of aerobic exercise outweigh the risks of cardiovascular disease as a result of long-term endurance training. However, for any one individual that may not be the case. There are runners who have had cardiac arrhythmias, high calcification scores for coronary arteries, and other unexpected cardiovascular problems. Of course, we do not have proof of cause and effect for these cases, but we think runners and endurance athletes should consult with their physicians and be serious consumers of forthcoming research on this topic.

Recent studies have challenged the long-held belief that endurance training provides protection against cardiovascular disease. We present results from these studies in Chapter 4. We are grateful to Michael S. Emery, MD, for providing his thoughts on these recent studies that have created concern among runners about the effects of long-term endurance training on heart health.

Runners get injured. That may be the singular drawback to the almost perfect physical activity. In Chapter 5, we are fortunate to share the advice and knowledge of D. S. Blaise Williams III, PhD.

Dr. Williams is a recognized expert on running injuries and gait analysis. His advice on how to avoid injuries is an important element in our effort to provide you with a plan for lifelong running.

Not being able to run can have serious health consequences. Once you become inactive, the beneficial aspects associated with aerobic physical activity are lost. Weight and waist size increase. Cholesterol and triglycerides increase. You lose stamina and muscle mass. We are attempting to provide a handbook for being a lifelong runner so you can maintain those healthy benefits associated with running and longevity.

We constantly read about new training programs and strategies. It can be confusing to figure out what might work for you. We lay out questions to ask for evaluating any training plan that you are considering. We emphasize in Chapter 6 that no one training plan is best. We are all unique individuals who respond differently to different types of training. There is a lot of trial and error that goes into finding what works best for you, and what works best at one time in your life may not be right at a later age.

In Chapter 7, we discuss the benefits of having a coach or training partner to provide an outside perspective on your training. The close relationships we have built through coaching are another valuable source of understanding how every runner is a unique subset of one.

No variable is more important to your training and racing than pacing. In Chapter 8, we offer advice on how to ensure that your training is effective and how smart pacing can optimize your race performance.

Nutrition is one of the most vexing health topics. Nutritional research studies are difficult to conduct. For health purposes, we are primarily interested in the long-term effects of dietary habits.

Those studies rely to a great extent on recall. There are serious limitations to one's ability to give an accurate account of food consumption over many years.

Similarly, determining the ideal nutritional plan for performance is quite difficult, if not impossible. Many variables affect performance. It is not easy to isolate the effect of nutrition. In Chapter 9, we discuss how the scientific community's nutritional recommendations have changed over the past 40 years. Even though nutrition is complicated, for good health, eating a healthy diet is simple.

"Diet is by far the most powerful intervention to delay aging and age-related diseases," according to Valter Longo, PhD, director of the University of Southern California's Longevity Institute. We make our general recommendations for putting together a healthy eating plan at the end of the chapter.

In Chapter 10, we offer advice on how to keep running in proper perspective. We want your running to be a joyful activity and not become drudgery. We offer our perspective on how to make your running fun and playful while pursuing your performance goals.

We aim to provide a sensible program to help you be healthy, fit, and fast for a lifetime. The 7-Hour Workout Week lays out the program in Chapter 11. This plan includes run workouts, cross-training workouts, strength (resistance) exercises, and stretches. However, we urge you to read the chapters that precede the plan itself to understand the principles that underlie the program.

In Chapter 12, even though we know that many runners resist this idea, we will try to convince you that strength training is an essential element in your quest to become a lifelong runner. It is also valuable for your current athletic performance. We chose exercises that will enhance your running and long-term health and show how to do them in detail.

In Chapter 13, we argue that stretching is an equally essential element in your quest to become a lifelong runner. We have chosen exercises that will enhance your running and increase the likelihood of maintaining flexibility as you age. Whatever else you might do to improve your health and fitness, do not neglect the recommendations to add regular strength training and stretching to your regimen.

All the information, training advice, and training plans are aimed at getting you fitter, faster, and healthier. To accomplish those goals and to continue strenuous activity as you age requires a balanced, comprehensive wellness approach to training. Health is more than just the absence of disease. It is a state of wellness that includes a balance of the primary dimensions of wellness—physical, mental, social, spiritual, and emotional. All of us are challenged to balance these wellness components.

What do we mean by "fit"? There are many definitions of fitness—some as general as being able to reproduce and survive in your environment and others as specific as being able to perform a set of detailed tasks. We consider fitness as a composite of cardio-respiratory fitness, muscular fitness, coordination, and balance.

"Fast" is a term relative to each individual. One runner might consider a 16-minute 5-K as fast while another thinks finishing under 40 minutes qualifies. By running fast, we mean having run workouts at 85 to 95 percent of your maximal oxygen consumption, being able to run hard for a 5-K, and training with the intention of fulfilling your potential and achieving your optimal performance. Running fast is an approach to your running that includes intentional hard efforts.

We recommend that runners of all ages include some high-intensity efforts in their training. We specify for you when and how that should be done. I still include hard, fast segments of running every week. No, not anywhere near the speed that I used to run, but the intensity is there and it feels fast. The training keeps me fit enough to jump into a race occasionally and not be crushed by the effort required. Scott and I still favor quality training over quantity.

If you are familiar with the running plans in *Run Less, Run Faster*, you will find one big difference in the 7-Hour Workout Week plans. The intensity for the run workouts is determined by your perceived level of effort rather than target times and paces. We are using this alternative method for establishing the required intensity for each workout for several reasons.

Runners often ask us for training plans when they are not training for specific races. For many runners, focusing on perceived effort reduces the stress levels that arise with striving to hit precise split times or paces. Runners can still maintain a high level of fitness by focusing on their exertion levels. A break from closely monitoring their watches will leave them refreshed and ready to begin the next race preparation cycle. They will still be fit and prepared when it is time to start a new 16-week training program for their next race.

Your form suffers when you are excessively focused on your watch. I have observed runners who check their GPS every 15 to 30 seconds to monitor their pace. This obsession prevents them from focusing on form and posture. Staring down all the time makes it impossible to maintain good running form with your head up looking forward. Furthermore, holding your wrist out to look at your watch constantly interrupts rhythmic arm movement. Obsessive pace monitoring is the enemy of good form and an efficient gait.

We want you to enjoy your running. Being mindful of your effort puts you more in tune with the running experience. Focusing on your effort, your breathing, your gait, and how you feel increases your awareness of the moment. You can improve your fitness with a good, hard effort and still have it be a relaxing experience.

You need to have a sense of pace. Runners who depend on their GPS to inform them of their pace fail to connect their effort with their pace. We suggest that you focus on perceived effort during your run. After the run, use the data from your watch as feedback information. That way you will learn to be in tune with your body and mind during the run, but you will be able to associate the effort with your pace. You may feel at sea initially, but this approach will lead to a genuine learning experience.

We realize that runners want to race. We also know that pace is important to goal achievement and success. For that reason, we have devoted a chapter to pacing later in the book, as well as an appendix section that provides information on paces that are equivalent to perceived levels of exertion.

Training to run a fast race time requires the expenditure of a lot of physical energy, which can contribute to stress and fatigue. Devoting a lot of your energy to physical training often leads to neglect of other aspects of your life. It is not uncommon for runners to report that they are happy to have a race done because of the stress brought on by their training. Finding the right type and amount of training is the key to maintaining running as a healthy, lifelong activity.

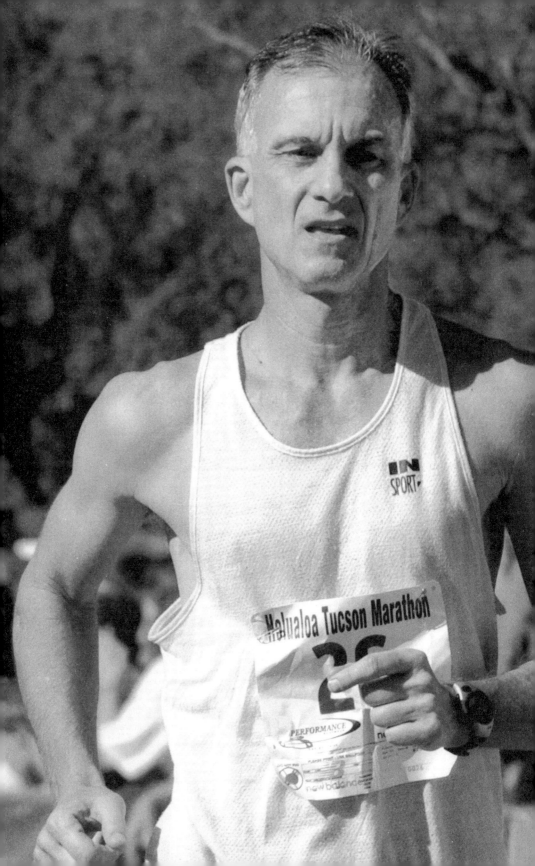

CHAPTER 1

WHAT HAS FIRST LEARNED FROM RUNNERS?

THE RUNNERS ARRIVED FROM NEW YORK, Washington State, Israel, Ohio, Texas, and Brazil, amongst other places. After they settled in at the local inn just a few minutes from Furman, we told them what they could expect over the next 4 days: lectures; classroom discussions; instructional demonstrations; hands-on participation in cross-training, strength training, and stretching sessions; and individual comprehensive laboratory assessments.

The next morning, these lawyers, physicians, professors, accountants, CEOs, and engineers filed nervously into the Molnar Human Performance Laboratory. All of these competent professionals were anxious about how they would perform on the treadmill and what the results might tell them about their fitness.

This scenario has been repeated at each of our Furman Institute of Running and Scientific Training (FIRST) Adult Running and Learning Retreats over the past 10 years. We have enjoyed and learned much through our interaction with participants from 40 states and more than 10 countries from Canada to India. A typical retreat class includes a few more males than females. The age of attendees has ranged from 23 to 79, with an average age of 48 and a range of 5-K race times from 17 to 40 minutes.

The retreat is designed to provide runners a positive and educational experience, and the knowledge we have gained about runners' habits, desires, strengths, weaknesses, and idiosyncrasies is immeasurable. Much of the basis for this book is a result of what we have learned about runners from our close association with retreat participants.

In 2007, FIRST offered its initial Running and Learning Retreat—a retreat, not a camp, because the emphasis is education, not training. In the 4-day retreat, the participants run only twice, not including the treadmill running on the first day of laboratory assessments. Our goal is to stimulate a love of running in adult athletes by sharing information about how to develop an effective training program, one that improves performance but also fosters sustainable running into old age.

The laboratory assessment includes aerobic capacity (VO_2 max), lactate threshold, body composition, and gait analysis. In the following paragraphs, we will detail the importance of each of these factors and the methods by which they are assessed. The limit of 16 participants ensures all can have an individual session with one or more of the retreat faculty to examine their test results and to discuss a plan for their future goals.

The running sessions concentrate on pacing for interval and tempo run training. We want the participants to focus on how the target time feels so they have a good sense of pace without staring at their watches. All participants leave the retreat with a personalized training plan that includes their personal target paces for each of their workouts.

What happens to the runner at the retreat does not need to stay at the retreat. At least, that is what we hope happens. The 12 runner profiles provided throughout the book are examples of how runners take home what they learn at the retreat and use it to change their training to avoid injuries, eliminate pain, and run faster. A typical example of how that happens is the story of John McCreesh IV.

John, a 45-year-old lawyer from Philadelphia, wanted to break 4 hours in the marathon. He recognized that his body type—a stocky 5 foot 7 inches and 195 pounds—was not ideal for distance running, but he enjoyed participating in races and wanted to have a goal to keep him focused.

John knew his successful legal practice got in the way of serious training and that his current lifestyle did not have him on a path to a healthy future. He needed a plan that would enable him to achieve his goals and that was compatible with his busy professional life. He came to us with hopes for finding a healthy blueprint.

On the first day of the 2012 FIRST retreat, John came into the Molnar Human Performance Laboratory, where Ray Moss put him on the treadmill, attached a face mask, and started him running. Every 4 minutes Ray increased the speed and John got a brief pause, but only long enough for Scott Murr to prick his finger to collect a drop of blood.

After several 4-minute stages, the data on the computer monitor told us that John was capable of another minute, though John might not have agreed. We wanted him to reach his max. So we encouraged him to keep going even when he wanted to quit. John, covered in sweat and slobber, completed the minute. We were assured from the data that showed his elevated ventilation, heart rate, respiratory exchange ratio, and blood lactate that he had maxed the test. John's panting and clinging to the treadmill railing left no doubt that he had given an all-out effort. These tests gave us the information needed to assess John's potential.

The reason we test for VO_2 max is to determine aerobic capacity, commonly referred to as the size of the runner's engine. It is a good indicator of overall potential.

The blood drawn every 4 minutes was placed in a lactate analyzer. Now we had the data to determine his lactate threshold, which is a particularly useful measure. It tells you how fast you can run before fatigue sets in. Both of these measures are fully explained later in the chapter.

We then shuttled John over to the biomechanics lab, where we videotaped his running to analyze his form for weaknesses. Many runners think they know if they pronate or supinate because they have been told so by a shoe salesperson. What we look for is whether there is any hip drop, torso twisting, foot crossover, hip-to-knee-to-footstrike relationship, and measured angles of push-off, recovery, and footstrike phases of gait. More discussion of gait analysis is provided later in this chapter.

Next, still sweaty from his treadmill workout, John got to lie down . . . on the bed of a dual-energy x-ray absorptiometry (DEXA) machine, which painlessly and unobtrusively scanned his whole body. Finally, a break. Until he got the results. Even though John looked fit enough, his body fat percentage categorized him near the top of the overweight category, just shy of obese. He was disheartened. John was carrying around extra weight that was not doing him any good. In many ways this is the hardest thing for runners to hear. And it is also the best news: Body composition is something you can address, unlike more fixed measures, such as your maximum heart rate and muscle fiber type. At last, we sat with him as he digested the results of his treadmill test, gait analysis, and body-composition figures.

Four days later, John returned to Philly armed with a training plan. He knew his optimal training pace (8:12/mile), that he would be wise to make smarter choices at the grocery store (trading in the chips for fruits) and at the deli (veggie sub instead of a cheesesteak), and that he needed to stop running so much and join a gym. We had taught him a series of strengthening and stretching exercises, and he realized how weak he was, and how inflexible. With all of these data, John knew a lot more about his level of fitness. Would it help him reach his goal of a faster half-marathon and a sub-4-hour marathon?

John's long-term commitment to the training plan paid dividends, though it took a while. Two years later he finished the New York City Marathon in 3:57, and four years later he finished the Chicago Marathon in 3:36.

John's cross-training, strength training, and improved diet contributed to a 28-pound weight loss and a much improved body composition. He was now fitter, faster, and healthier.

Just as we did with John, we meet with each runner to learn about his or her goals. We discuss participants' training and the challenges they face. Before they leave the retreat, we develop a plan to help them attain their goals.

Like John, many of the runners who attend the retreats are middle-aged professionals. We get men and women who come with a wide range of talent. They are focused on distances from 5-K to the marathon. Many come looking to overcome a series of injuries. Some are seeking something extra to achieve a personal best or to qualify for Boston. Most say they want to be running for many years to come.

Why Should You Get Tested in the Lab?

As discussed above, the factor, or factors, that a runner can improve can be determined with laboratory testing. Lab testing can accurately measure a runner's current level of fitness as well as identify appropriate training and racing paces and the runner's optimal body weight. According to the research literature, by knowing their VO_2 max, lactate threshold, running economy, and body composition, runners (or their coaches) will have the necessary information to determine what changes in training are appropriate.[1] Repeat testing can confirm whether or not the elements of a training program are effective and indicate needed modifications.

Estimates of VO_2 max, lactate threshold, and body composition by speed/distance monitors or smartphone apps are just that: estimates. Given the known inaccuracies associated with such estimates, it is preferable that runners base their training on accurate measurements from lab testing.

We recommend that runners look for a camp or clinic that provides a comprehensive physiological and biomechanical laboratory assessment. You may find those services at a local university, hospital, or running-performance center. John's experience is typical of what occurs in a laboratory assessment. Let us look more closely at the important laboratory measures that can tell you a lot about your fitness. This information can be applied to improve your training plan.

The Laboratory Measures Defined
Maximal Oxygen Consumption (VO_2 max)

It is common for articles about elite runners to refer to their VO_2 max and how it compares to that of other current and past runners. Serious runners are more likely to know the late Steve Prefontaine's VO_2 max score than his best 5-K time or how his score compares with Frank Shorter's or Jim Ryun's. It is a key measurement of endurance running ability and a good indicator of one's potential as a runner.

We are always intrigued with athletes who have extraordinary physical characteristics. When it comes to endurance athletes, it is VO_2 max that we use to describe the extraordinarily talented, just as we use vertical jump to describe the special talent of a basketball player. My wonderful parents failed to provide me with either a big, aerobic engine or the ability to soar above the basket, but they imparted a love of participation.

Maximal oxygen consumption (VO_2 max) is the maximum amount of oxygen the body can utilize during exercise. Muscles need oxygen to produce energy efficiently. That means having a strong heart and vascular system that can pump blood and deliver it to the working muscles. The muscles' ability to extract and utilize that oxygen is equally as important. VO_2 max, which is largely determined by genetics, can be improved with training; for untrained individuals, VO_2 max can be improved by as much as 20 percent.[2]

There is a strong relationship between VO_2 max and performance capabilities. The higher your maximal oxygen uptake, the more oxygen you can deliver to your muscles and the more energy you can produce, enabling you to work harder or run faster.

VO_2 max for runners is determined in the laboratory by testing the runner on a treadmill using a strict protocol. The protocol includes stages at specific speeds, with the speed systematically increased for each new stage. The volume and concentration of oxygen inhaled and exhaled are measured to determine the amount of oxygen consumed during each stage.

As the treadmill speed increases and the workload is greater, the oxygen consumption increases. When the speed and workload increase but the runner's consumption of oxygen does not increase to satisfy the increased demand, the amount of oxygen consumed at that moment is known as the runner's VO_2 max. For a valid test, the runner must give an all-out effort. Knowing your VO_2 max by itself alone is only one piece of the puzzle. Another part of the performance puzzle is how effectively your body is able to use the available oxygen. That is where our second laboratory measure, lactate threshold, comes into play.

Among runners with the same VO_2 max, there will be a wide spread in their finish times. While elite runners do indeed have similar VO_2 max values, the runner with the highest VO_2 max is not always the first to cross the finish line.

Lactate Threshold

Lactate threshold essentially defines the upper limit of sustainable efforts in training and racing. If VO_2 max can be seen as an upper limit for aerobic exercise, then lactate threshold determines how much of that aerobic upper limit can be used over a sustained period of effort. When lactate threshold improves, endurance running performance improves.[3]

Endurance events are not run at 100 percent of VO_2 max. In general, the percentage of VO_2 max that runners can maintain during a race is determined by their lactate thresholds. It is a measure of the body's maximal steady-state exercise capacity.

Lactate threshold is most commonly defined as the exercise intensity that produces blood lactate faster than the body can clear it. Even when you are walking down the street, your body produces lactate. As your exercise intensity increases, your lactate production increases. As long as the body is able to clear it by shuttling it within the cell and to other working muscles and the liver, the blood lactate levels stay low. Once the intensity reaches a point where the lactate cannot be shuttled to be used as a fuel, it hinders muscular contraction and leads to fatigue.

Whether we are talking about lactate threshold or lactic acid threshold, the difference is largely a matter of semantics (the difference between lactate and lactic acid is chemical; when lactic acid enters the blood, it drops a hydrogen ion and becomes lactate). Thus, the more appropriate term is lactate threshold.

As blood lactate accumulates, the muscles' ability to contract declines. The reduced muscular contraction decreases the amount of work the muscles can produce, thus resulting in slower running. A runner's lactate threshold can be improved with training.

There are methods for estimating lactate threshold that do not include taking blood samples. Trained runners can use their 10-K race pace as a good ballpark estimate of their lactate threshold pace.

However, the most accurate method for determining lactate threshold is by completing an exercise test that uses a defined protocol in a laboratory setting. The test is usually conducted on a treadmill where speed and elevation can be controlled precisely. During a lactate threshold test, the speed of the treadmill is increased at regular intervals (e.g., every 3 to 4 minutes), and blood samples by finger prick are taken at each stage. The test begins at an easy effort level, and each stage gets progressively faster or harder. At the end of each stage, a small sample of blood is collected to measure blood lactate. Typically runners will have their fingers pricked six to nine times during a test to measure the level of lactate in the blood.

The data from the treadmill are examined to see where the lactate level increased significantly. The runner's speed at which the lactate began accumulating sharply is determined to be the lactate threshold running speed. This speed is where the runner will want to concentrate much of her or his training.

The goal of training at or near the lactate threshold pace is to enable the body to adapt by raising the lactate threshold. That is, a greater lactate threshold means that you can run at a faster steady-state speed without a sharp rise in the accumulation of lactate. You will be able to run at a greater percentage of your VO_2 max for a longer time.

Running Speed at VO_2 max (vVO_2 max)

Great laboratory data may be something to take pride in or to brag about with friends, but what really matters when it comes to race day is how fast you are. A better measure of fitness, which takes efficiency into account, is how fast athletes are running when they hit their VO_2 max.

Running speed or velocity at VO_2 max (vVO_2 max) is the running speed that produces the highest-possible rate of oxygen consumption.[4] Typically this is measured by a lab test. In fact vVO_2 max is considered to be the best predictor of endurance running performance since it integrates both aerobic capacity (VO_2 max) and running economy.[5]

Running speed at VO_2 max can be used to explain the differences in race performance between two runners of equal VO_2 max or running economy. If two runners have the same VO_2 max values or have a similar economy of motion, then the runner with the higher vVO_2 max will be running at a faster speed for any given percentage of his or her VO_2 max. Improvements in vVO_2 max translate to improved running performance. Most runners are able to improve their vVO_2 max.

Running at vVO_2 max increases leg strength, and enhanced strength tends to result in improved running economy. The muscles are stronger, thus the energy cost is lower. vVO_2 max efforts improve neuromuscular fitness, which reduces energy expenditure.[6]

Body Composition

Body composition is used to describe an individual's percentages of fat and nonfat tissue. The nonfat, or lean, tissue consists of bone, fluid, muscle, and organs. Muscle is more metabolically active than fat and raises the resting metabolic rate. Fat is used for storing calories and has a low energy demand, meaning it does not burn many calories.

Given the role of fat tissue in regulating blood lipids and insulin insensitivity, it is important that body composition be monitored in the management of one's health. Too much fat tissue can undermine one's health.

Body weight is not necessarily a good indicator of body composition. You can be overfat but not overweight, because you have little lean muscle. You can also be very muscular with a low percentage of body fat, but you might be considered overweight by medical and insurance tables because of your size. That is why defining measures of body composition are more important than body weight.

Excess body fat increases one's body weight without contributing to the body's capacity to utilize oxygen. As a result, a high body fat percentage lowers VO_2 max. Excess body fat affects running performance by lowering the energy available for running.

Body composition is not only an important performance factor but a key component of fitness and overall health. The accurate assessment of body composition is valuable information for anyone wishing to be healthy, fit, and fast. We find that most runners attending our retreats are surprised to learn that their body composition numbers are not as favorable as they had expected.

There are numerous methods for assessing body composition. A brief description follows, with comments on the accuracy, advantages, and disadvantages of each method. The most basic methods of estimating body composition are anthropometric measures, including skinfold measurements, abdominal circumference, and body mass index (BMI).

Skinfold measurements typically are taken at three to seven different sites around the body. The technician pinches the skin to raise a double layer of skin and the underlying adipose tissue and records the thickness using calipers. While skinfold measurement does provide regional body fat assessment, this method of assessing body composition does not measure deep belly fat, an important factor in terms of health.

BMI is determined by calculating a ratio of weight to height. A high BMI can be an indicator of high body fatness. However, BMI can be misleading because it is not a measure of excess fat. It is a popular and quick method for estimating one's weight category. It can incorrectly categorize those who are especially muscular as overweight. Of greater concern is that those who are categorized as normal weight may be overfat and at risk of heart disease and diabetes. There are other metrics that do a much better job of identifying these people—all we have to do is measure some hips and waists.

Measuring the abdominal circumference is a quick and easy method for assessing belly fat. An association between excess abdominal fat and various health risks has been identified. Waist-to-hip ratio is another indicator of excess abdominal fat. The ratio should be less than 0.94 for men and less than 0.85 for women.[7]

Underwater weighing was once used almost exclusively for determining body composition. However, electronic methods have largely supplanted its use. Subjects being tested by underwater weighing must expel all the air from their lungs and, while completely submerged, remain perfectly still so that an underwater weight can be recorded. Besides needing a tank and equipment to conduct the test, many subjects are not comfortable with exhaling their air and staying submerged until a measure is obtained.

Today, it is becoming more common for most fitness centers to use bioelectrical impedance analysis (BIA) for predicting body fat because the equipment is not very expensive and the operator does not require special training. BIA is based on the principle that an electric signal travels through the body at different rates depending upon the body's composition. The proportion of body fat can be calculated since the signal travels more easily through the parts of the body that are composed mostly of water (e.g., body fluids, muscle) than it does through bone, fat, or air. BIA is not very accurate for very heavy and very light individuals. A shortcoming with the BIA is that many of the devices do not measure belly fat.

DEXA, used primarily for bone density testing, is considered the preferred method for body composition testing. Since different types of body tissue absorb an x-ray energy beam at different rates, the machine can distinguish between bone mineral content, lean mass, and fat mass. The scan involves having an individual lie faceup on a table as the machine makes a 6- to 12-minute single pass over the body. The procedure is totally painless, and the results are immediate.

Bod Pod is another popular method used to assess body composition. Bod Pod determines body composition (fat mass versus lean mass) in a manner similar in principle to underwater weighing by measuring the volume of air displaced by the body while the individual sits in a large, egg-shaped chamber instead of a tank of water. Using computerized pressure sensors to determine the amount of air displaced by the body, the measurements can be taken in about 10 minutes.

At FIRST, we use both DEXA and Bod Pod for determining body composition. Both are fast and accurate. DEXA provides more details about the body's fat-distribution pattern. The disadvantages are that both methods use expensive equipment that may not be easily accessible in many locations.

Gait Analysis

Why should you get a gait analysis? A gait analysis is for runners who want to improve their running mechanics, their running economy, and thereby their performance, and for runners who have recurring running-related injuries.

Faulty running mechanics reduce efficiency and usually result in excessive stress on the lower extremities and pelvis, which increases the likelihood of an injury. A gait analysis discovers inefficiencies and the compensations a runner makes. Each runner's gait is unique.

In addition to increasing the risk of injury, unnecessary, improper, and unbalanced movements limit a runner's potential. Unless the underlying causes of dysfunctional movement patterns are addressed, a runner's movement patterns will not change, and, unfortunately, the risk of injury will not be reduced. So for runners who keep getting injured even though they are otherwise healthy, a gait analysis can be valuable.

Running economy is the energy cost of running at a specific intensity. Two runners can have the same VO_2 max and the same lactate threshold yet one may be superior in races. The runner with a better running economy uses less energy (i.e., consumes less oxygen) at a given pace. Running economy, for that reason, is a better predictor of performance than VO_2 max.

We can store only a certain amount of fuel in the working muscles to be used for running. If we become more economical, then our fuel storage will last longer—assuming that we are running at the same speed.

The good news is that running economy can be improved with training. Developing the ability to absorb the energy from the shock of landing and transferring that to push-off is a key biomechanical factor in becoming more economical. Also, runners become more economical when they learn to improve muscle activation. Performing a variety of workouts at different distances and intensities enhances our muscle-fiber-recruitment pattern and the ability to recruit more muscle mass. That makes the runner more economical and helps delay fatigue.

When training for a specific race, a good training program will include training segments at race pace as a means to become more economical at that specific speed. Also, fast running will contribute to improving running economy.

Biomechanics influence running economy, too. Videotaping a runner on a treadmill is a technique used for assessing a runner's gait. A trained analyst can determine whether a runner overstrides, uses the arms ineffectively, or has too much head movement for optimal efficiency, for example.

The analysis typically begins with runners' providing information on their current training, goals, and injury history. Initially conducted on an examination table, the gait analysis includes body measurements, range-of-motion measurements, and a series of movements to evaluate a runner's flexibility, balance, and strength. A running session on a treadmill videotaped from different angles typically follows. A meaningful gait analysis is much more elaborate than having a shoe salesperson eyeball your running on an in-store treadmill.

It is common that inefficient gaits, muscular weaknesses, and flexibility issues are revealed in the gait analyses conducted on our retreat participants. I tell them that the recommendations they are given as a result of the analysis could easily be well worth the expense and time for attending the retreat. For many, following our recommendations has meant faster running and the elimination of chronic injuries. Those recommendations typically include specific strengthening and stretching exercises.

Runners typically become more economical with years of training. The body adapts to accommodate the demands placed on it over time. Consistent, sustained training has its benefits and, perhaps, none more valuable than increased running economy.

How Can the Lab Data Be Used to Enhance My Running?

Five years ago, Furman University hired Robert Gary to direct its cross-country and track-and-field program. Coach Gary, a six-time All-American and Big Ten Champion at Ohio State University and an Olympian, competed in the 3000-meter steeplechase at the 1996 Olympics in Atlanta and the 2004 Games in Athens. He immediately elevated the success of Furman's distance running program. Both the men's and women's cross-country teams won Southern Conference championships in his second, third, and fourth seasons at the helm. The men's cross-country team also finished 13th in the Division I NCAA National Cross-Country Championships in his third year as coach.

Coach Gary is a strong believer in the value of laboratory assessments. He contends that the development of outstanding runners requires that both the art and science of coaching be applied to create each competitor's training. Before he even joined us at Furman, he came to us at FIRST and asked if we could provide laboratory assessments for his runners. We have assessed his runners with all the tests mentioned above. Since his arrival at Furman, we have tested all the runners at the beginning of the year as well at the end of the season. He not only has data to design their workouts, he can also track their progress over 4 years.

In particular, Coach Gary requests a gait analysis on his runners who have an injury or an apparent gait abnormality. It is valuable for runners to view their running in slow motion with commentary describing their inefficiencies.

We use the data similarly in providing each FIRST retreat participant with an individualized training plan. For those who need a boost in VO_2 max, we include track repeat workouts with a focus on higher-intensity training and a recommendation to attain ideal body weight. For those whose lactate threshold is limiting their running, we include tempo runs at specific paces identified during the treadmill test. We also address the improvement of running economy by including exercises to increase strength and power, which contribute to better running form and efficiency.

Many of the runners we have observed at our retreats share common traits. Here is what we have learned about runners over 10 years of conducting retreats.

Runners Tend To:

Find an Identity in Running

Even though many runners are talented and successful professionals with a wide range of interests and community involvements, they embrace an identity as a runner. They are apt to have a 26.2 or 13.1 sticker on their cars or a personalized license plate such as LUV2RUN. They proudly wear their latest race T-shirt. They write accounts of their latest running accomplishments for the local newspaper, running-club newsletter, or blog. They celebrate with friends on social media and inspire others to set goals. They also travel as a group to races.

This is because they are dedicated. All of us value accomplishments that are difficult and require strenuous efforts spread over many weeks. Race success does not come from a few days of training. Running success is typically the result of months and years of dedication. This dedication includes overcoming heat, cold, rain, illnesses, injuries, fatigue, and rising early on weekend mornings for that essential long training run.

Running, like other sports, provides a clear result. You can see the outcome of your efforts. It is part of the appeal of sports. That is not always true in other aspects of life, where you may not know for years, if ever, the outcome of your dedication and conscientious efforts.

That is why runners often describe their finish-line emotions with phrases such as "best day of my life," "a dream come true," and "thrill of a lifetime."

Be Motivated by Specific Goals

Most runners have a lengthy list of goals. Whether it is to run faster, farther, or a certain number of races, these short-term and long-term goals dictate future training and racing. Runners commonly report that they enjoy training much more, and are likely to be more compliant with their training plans, when the training is focused on a specific race goal.

These goals are powerful. They influence daily habits, vacation plans, social lives, and participation in other recreational activities and interests.

Want to Achieve Those Goals Now

While serious runners tend to be disciplined and hardworking, they often need to learn patience. Because rapid improvement comes easily to neophyte runners, they come to expect those PRs to continue and are often disappointed when they realize that the law of diminishing returns applies to fitness. As they approach their potential, they learn that it will take a lot of hard training to improve a small amount. Setting a goal of qualifying for Boston soon after your first 5-K is a setup for failure.

Often Pursue Conflicting Goals

We receive many messages from runners asking how to adapt their training to enable them to run a 5-K, then 2 weeks later compete in a triathlon, and 2 weeks after that run a marathon. As one of my colleagues likes to say, "The hunter who chases two rabbits catches none." That analogy definitely applies to training for races of different distances.

Training is goal specific. The training needed for a fast 5-K is different from the training necessary for racing 26.2 miles.

One problem is that runners do not get the full benefits of their training programs because they disrupt a carefully developed training regimen with frequent racing that requires tapering and recoveries. Many cannot resist the urge to race long enough to focus on training for a singular event. One race in the middle of a training plan provides feedback on current fitness and race goals. Multiple races during the training cycle tend to detract from the plan's benefits.

We counsel runners to focus fully on one goal at a time. Later they may be able to capitalize on the benefits of the training for that goal to enhance the training for their next goal.

Always Be at Risk of Injury

Throughout the chapters in this book, we address injuries. That is because they are a major issue for runners. We caution runners that as they fine-tune their fitness, they are more vulnerable to injury. Most training programs intersperse weeks of reduced training to allow the body to recover from the cumulative stress.

Runners' desire to get faster can lead to their ignoring rest and recovery. It is easy to undermine good efforts by constantly increasing training volume and intensity.

Ignore Early Signs of a Potential Injury

It is far too common for us to hear from runners that they have been dealing with a soreness, irritation, and/or pain for a long time. They will try to run through it rather than seek treatment as soon as it is detected. As a result, the inflammation gets worse. The sad truth is, if you do not treat a problem early, you are in for a prolonged rehabilitation and time away from running.

Not Cross-Train Consistently or Effectively

Frequently runners who claim to have followed the FIRST program write to us saying it did not work. They missed their goal marathon time by 90 seconds. When we ask about their training, many confess that while they did every run at exactly the pace specified, they did not do any of the cross-training. Our "3plus2" training program is just that: three quality runs *plus* two cross-training workouts each week. The cross-training is as important as the running if you want to reach your goal time.

Cross-training, as we describe in Chapter 11, has significant benefits—improved fitness while reducing the likelihood of injury—if done properly.

Benefit from Coaching Assistance

In Chapter 7, we describe the benefits of coaching. We have observed that runners with coaches benefit from having their own individualized plans. They also are aided by having someone monitor their activities and detect when their training needs to be modified. Having a coach adds accountability and an incentive to follow the plan as designed.

UP CLOSE AND PERSONAL

Lorie is a triathlete. First, she was a competitive swimmer who took up biking to ride with friends. Finally, she added running to her training. She reports that she rarely goes a day without a morning run, bike, or swim. She clearly enjoys all three disciplines.

Here is how Lorie describes the development of her running and why she enjoys it.

Name: Lorie Tucker

Age: 49

Occupation: USAT Certified Triathlon Coach

Hometown: Mesa, AZ

Race times: Utah Valley Marathon, 3:50; Ironman Florida, 12:15

Age she began running: 36

- I was an observer for many years while my husband ran marathons and competed in local 10-Ks and charity races.
- I began with 5-Ks, then 10-Ks, halfs, and then full marathons. And I had the time of my life doing relays like Ragnar in various states and locations.
- Running is such a pure and amazing experience. I love the simplicity of pulling on my shoes and hitting the road.
- But like every competitive person out there, I wanted to be faster. I wanted to improve. I jumped at the opportunity to improve myself and gain knowledge, not only for myself but so I could coach others on how to be faster without putting in 70 to 80 miles per week solely running.
- Nutrition, gait analysis, and cross-training all enhanced my understanding of how to train more effectively.

As a triathlon coach, Lorie came to the retreat hungry to learn the subtle and nuanced aspects of training. She asked lots of questions and took lots of notes. She embodies the notion that a smarter runner will be a better runner.

Not Train or Race at the Right Pace

All runners have suffered at one time from training or racing at the wrong pace, either too slow or too fast. If you run too slowly in training, your body will not be able to adapt to the need for greater fitness. When your training runs are too fast, you may not be able to complete the workout, or your fatigue will undermine the next few workouts.

In a race, if the pace is too slow, it is obvious you will not hit your goal time. If the pace is too fast, well, we all know how that story ends. It can be a long, miserable march to the finish line.

We are surprised by how many runners who attend our retreats do not know their appropriate training paces, even though they tell us that they do track repeats and tempo runs regularly. Runners need to know those paces and have a good feel for them even without the use of a watch.

Neglect the Development of Good Flexibility

We regularly hear, "I know I should stretch, but I just do not have the time." We want to convince you that you do not have the time *not* to stretch, at least if you want to continue running into your forties and beyond. As we age, we lose flexibility. This shows up in gait analyses, where we see tight hamstrings, poor ankle flexibility, and tight hip flexors among other elements of poor posture.

Not Work on Improving Their Form, Posture, and Gait

At FIRST, we frequently identify poor running form as a weakness of our retreat attendees. Their running posture is poor because of muscular weaknesses, poor flexibility, and a lack of focus on form. We strive to provide training to improve their poor posture and, in doing so, prevent and remedy injuries.

Common postural problems include hip drop upon footstrike, which is a result of weak gluteal muscles. Strengthening the gluteal muscles is important for addressing this deficiency. Tight hip flexors restrict the knee-drive phase of the gait cycle. Regularly stretching the hip flexors is necessary for runners.

Often Sabotage Their Efforts with Unnecessary and Extra Weight

Over and over, we encounter runners who are dedicated to and disciplined in their training and determined to achieve their goals. What prevents them from achieving their goals is simply the extra weight they are carrying. The same dietary challenges contributing to America's obesity epidemic are common to runners, even if they look fit.

Developing and attaining a healthy eating plan is a major challenge for everyone, but it is especially true for runners who want to improve. Some runners still like to say that they run so they can eat what they want. You can do this. But you probably will not achieve your goals.

Want to Qualify for Boston

Without a doubt, the most common immediate goal we hear from runners, whether their most recent marathon time is 5 minutes short of qualification, an hour short of qualification, or whether they have never run more than a 5-K, is to qualify to run the Boston Marathon. They want us to tell them if they can do *it*.

We can use their training data and race times to predict a finish time and indicate whether their goal is realistic. It sometimes means that the goal needs to be set into the future by a year or two. In the meantime, intermediate goals—for example, a specific half-marathon race time—need to be established that will lead to that all-important qualifying time.

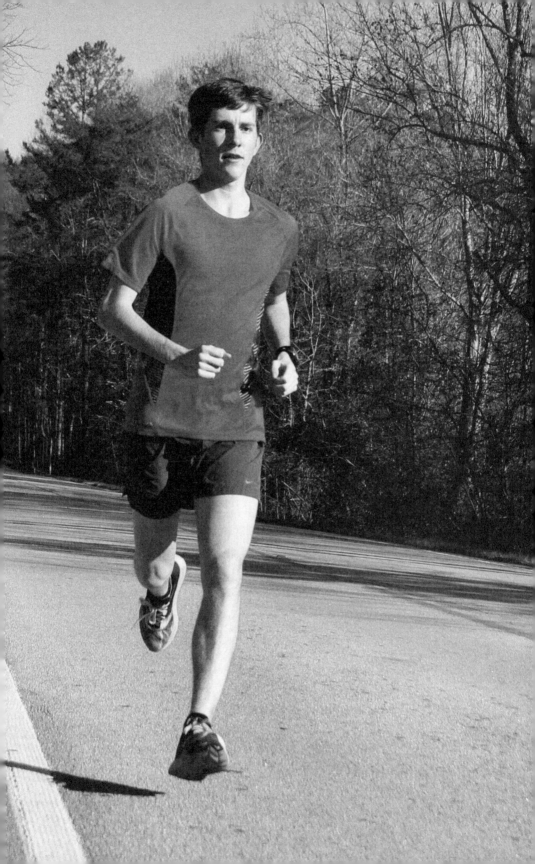

CHAPTER **2**

HOW CAN I RUN INTO OLD AGE?

IN RECENT YEARS, MOST CONVERSATIONS with my brother, Don, and colleague Scott come around to how our running is affected by aging. Scott is just approaching that mid-fifties age range where data show that a significant impact on performance begins to occur. Don and I are at that second aging checkpoint—mid- to late sixties—where the aging effects accelerate.

Our goal, like that of so many aging runners, is to be able to keep doing what we love to do. So we ask ourselves, What are the roadblocks to running immortality? What can we do now to increase the likelihood of being able to run for a lot longer? That is really what this book is all about. For you and for us.

We developed the 7-Hour Workout Week plan for ourselves, because we believe it is the smart way to offset our physical challenges. We know that the challenges associated with physiological, neurological, orthopedic, and biomechanical deterioration pose a threat to the longevity of a running career. How can we all avoid becoming ex-runners?

Over the past 50 years of competitive running, I have observed many runners and their running careers. Unfortunately, many were not able to continue running, even though it had been a central and important part of their lives. How can the large group of 40-year-olds running today still be running in the next 20 to 30 years?

At FIRST, we hear not only from runners who want to improve but also from former runners who have given up. There are many types of ex-runners. One is the person who trains daily and races often. This runner never does strength training, cross-training, or stretching. She is talented and wins or places in her age group in a lot of local races. She receives tons of reinforcement for her performances, so she tries not to let anything interfere with her training. She is genetically lucky enough to tolerate a high volume of training and frequent intense racing.

At the first sign of injury, which often occurs in the early to mid-forties, she keeps training. When the injury gets so bad that she must seek treatment, she does just enough rehabilitation to be able to get back on the road and immediately tries to make up for lost training, which only exacerbates the source of the injury. Then she enters a cycle of rehab, interspersed with striving to regain her peak conditioning, until she must stop training for a long period of recovery. This sequence may stretch over months or even years. Eventually, frustration wins out, and the superb performer becomes an ex-runner.

Another potential ex-runner is one who continues to train but who also loves to eat. While that was not a problem in his twenties or thirties, a few extra pounds per year has started to accumulate, and soon he has a spare tire around his middle. Over a decade of constant weight gain, he finds it difficult to train and race with an extra 15 to 25 pounds. After several unsuccessful attempts to lose weight and maintain the loss, he gives up and retires to the couch.

Because aging runners generally reduce their amount of training, it becomes unclear to what extent the slower race times are a result of aging or just less training. Aging runners are susceptible to injuries that can interrupt training. There might also be psychological and cultural factors that lead to either less training or lower-quality training. These are the aging running issues we will address in this chapter. While we may not be able to definitively clarify all of these issues, the slower race times associated with aging are well documented.

We know we will get slower as we age. What can we do to minimize the slowing?

We will provide advice about how to counter the factors that lead to becoming an ex-runner. We envision this book as becoming a handbook for lifelong running.

Do Aging Runners Continue to Participate in Races?

Since most of the people who come to the FIRST retreats are over 40, and many are over 50, we often hear them say, "I want to still be running when I reach 80" or "I never plan to stop running." Our participants tend to prioritize running, and in that at least, they may be unusual. The number of people who race begins to decline at age 50, and the falloff increases with each subsequent 5-year age group.

The tables on page 28 display the number of male and female finishers for the 2014 New York City Marathon[1] and the 2015 Peachtree Road Race,[2] the two largest road races in the country.

2014 New York City Marathon Finishers by Age Group

AGE GROUP	MALE FINISHERS	% OF MALES	FEMALE FINISHERS	% OF FEMALES
20–24	636	2.12%	746	3.67%
25–29	2,407	8.04%	2,985	14.68%
30–34	4,139	13.83%	3,738	18.38%
35–39	4,935	16.48%	3,381	16.62%
40–44	5,883	19.65%	3,536	17.39%
45–49	4,624	15.45%	2,647	13.01%
50–54	3,758	12.55%	1,831	9.00%
55–59	1,896	6.33%	898	4.42%
60–64	1,045	3.49%	402	1.98%
65–69	414	1.38%	121	0.59%
70–74	152	0.51%	43	0.21%
75–79	38	0.13%	9	0.04%
80–89	10	0.03%	2	0.01%
	29,937		20,339	

2015 Peachtree Road Race 10-K Finishers by Age Group

AGE GROUP	MALE FINISHERS	% OF MALES	FEMALE FINISHERS	% OF FEMALES
20–24	1,426	4.76%	1,891	9.30%
25–29	2,359	7.88%	3,031	14.90%
30–34	2,764	9.23%	3,374	16.59%
35–39	2,862	9.56%	3,421	16.82%
40–44	3,209	10.72%	3,495	17.18%
45–49	3,219	10.75%	3,193	15.70%
50–54	3,129	10.45%	2,803	13.78%
55–59	2,286	7.64%	2,007	9.87%
60–64	1,614	5.39%	1,168	5.74%
65–69	1,036	3.46%	543	2.67%
70–74	449	1.50%	160	0.79%
75–79	140	0.47%	44	0.22%
80–89	50	0.17%	12	0.06%
	24,543		25,142	

For both females and males, the participation in these two road races increased steadily from age 20 and peaked around 40 years old. Participation began to decline around age 45. The rate of decline in participation accelerated at age 55 and again at 65.

When Does Aging Make a Big Difference in Participation?

The table below shows that in both the 1995 and 2014 New York City Marathons, there was a significant drop-off in participation for both males and females from the 50–54 age group to the 55–59 age group. Even today, only half of the men and women in the 50–54 age group continue to participate into the 55–59 age group.

Comparison of Participation of Men's and Women's 50-54 and 55-59 Age Groups in 1995 and 2014 New York City Marathons

1995				
AGE GROUP	MEN	% MEN	WOMEN	% WOMEN
50–54	1,769	65.0%	330	71.6%
55–59	951	35.0%	131	28.4%
TOTAL	2,720		461	

2014				
AGE GROUP	MEN	% MEN	WOMEN	% WOMEN
50–54	3,758	66.5%	1,831	67.1%
55–59	1,896	33.5%	898	32.9%
TOTAL	5,654		2,729	

Ratio of Male Participation 2014 vs. 1996	2.1 to 1
Ratio of Female Participation 2014 vs. 1997	5.9 to 1

What causes this reduction in participation as runners age? First, let us look at some of the research findings on the effects of aging on running performance.

What Happens to Performance?

Runners slow with age, generally beginning around 35 years old. In the table below and on page 31, graphs show the fifth-place female and male single-age finish times from the 2015 New York City Marathon.[3] The graphs illustrate that the slower marathon finish times increase gradually from 35 to 55 and increase at a slightly faster rate from 55 to 65; after 65, the annual slowing becomes significantly greater. As with participation, aging begins to have a significant effect at age 55.

We chose the fifth-place finisher for every single age to represent that age, rather than the first-place finisher because the first-place finisher is often an outlier and not representative of that age. We assumed that the fifth-place finisher in each age group in the largest and one of the most prestigious marathons in the world represented a runner who trains seriously. For that reason, the time differences among these runners could be attributed primarily to the effects of aging.

New York City Marathon 2015
Fifth Place Female Finish Times by Age

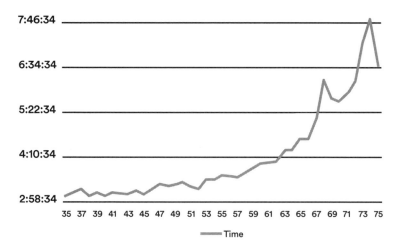

New York City Marathon 2015
Fifth Place Male Finish Times by Age

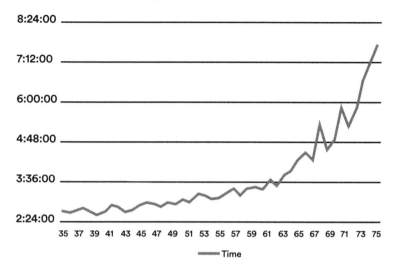

— Time

What Can You Expect to Happen to Your Running as You Age?

Once you hit 40, you are unlikely to get any faster. Unless, of course, you did not start running until you were, like a fine wine, already nicely mature. We have had runners at the Furman running retreats who have run personal bests in their late sixties. They did not begin running until their early sixties. Their performances confirm that it is possible to continue improving even at an age where biological aging is accelerated, which shows it is never too late to begin an exercise program.

Even though it is not uncommon for masters runners to win local road races, elite endurance athletes tend to slow in their mid- to late thirties.

Runners who remain fit and avoid serious injury can expect to see approximately 0.5 to 1 percent decline in performance per year from age 35 to 60. That means that if you are running a 20-minute 5-K at age 40, your 5-K time will be closer to 23 minutes by age 60.

It depends on whether you are willing and able to maintain the training volume and intensity of your younger years. As we age, we face physiological changes, such as loss of muscle mass, and orthopedic ones, like a reduced range of motion. And of course we all struggle with time and motivation.

Those who attend our FIRST retreats often say that they find it more difficult to sustain training intensity, that they need more time for recovery, and that their figures are no longer as girlish and boyish as they once were. Given this, we would expect to see their performances suffer.

Most of us begin to slow down after the age of 40 because our aerobic capacity is no longer what it was—we lose about 10 percent of our VO_2 max each decade we age—and we are more likely both to get injured and to need more time to heal than in years past.

It is the natural order. We age. Our senses become less acute, and we borrow each other's reading glasses in restaurants. We ask our kids and colleagues to repeat themselves. We might groan a little when we bend down to pick up the newspaper. But while we cannot hold back the tide, we can learn to surf. Fitness can help postpone the ill effects of aging, and while it will not make you immortal, it can prolong your life.

What Biological Changes Affect Your Running?

As we age, various indignities and infelicities are inflicted on our bodies. We lose muscle mass and bone density, causing us to shrink and shrivel, even as we pad ourselves with a layer of fat. Various changes lead to a loss of function.

Physiological changes that influence running and physical activity performance include:

> Reduced lean muscle mass

> Reduced bone mineral density

> Increased body fat

> Reduced cardiac output

> Reduced metabolic rate

> Hormonal changes[4]

As a basketball player, at 30 my quickness and reaction time were a bit slower than in my competitive collegiate days, and my loss of fast-twitch muscle fibers kept me closer to the ground, though I could still compete with the college players into my forties. I lost that ability in my fifties. In tennis, basketball, track (sprinting and jumping events), and football (running backs and receivers), it is hard to be a superstar after the age of 30.

But how does biological aging impact endurance running performance?

The main factor that affects us as we age is our ability to supply oxygen to the working muscles as we once could. Most researchers have chosen to focus on measurements of VO_2 max in order to investigate how physiological factors limit running performance as an athlete ages.

Through vigorous training you can reduce the loss of VO_2 max from the standard 10 percent per decade for couch potatoes to about 5 percent per decade between the ages of 35 and 60.[5] A dedication to staying fit is necessary to keep that fist-sized organ pumping strong.

As we age, we lose the ability to raise our heart rate to its previous maximum level, even with the most intense exercise. This reduction in maximal heart rate is inevitable and is what leads to the decline in cardiac output and VO_2 max. There are other factors—slight reductions in stroke volume and peripheral extraction, which can be maintained at relatively high levels with vigorous training—but these have less effect on our aerobic capacity.

As a runner ages, the other two important factors in running performance—lactate threshold and running economy—are not affected as much as maximal oxygen uptake. In fact, studies show that older runners who continue to train at high intensity are able to perform at a higher percentage of their VO_2 max than younger runners. Improvements in running economy often offset some of the declines in maximal oxygen uptake that normally occur with aging.

Our hearts and lungs are not the only body parts that influence performance. Connective tissues between the muscles and bones become more rigid as we age, and our tendons, ligaments, and joint capsules become less elastic.[6] These changes can restrict our range of movement and contribute to injuries. If our stride length is restricted, we will not be able to cover as much ground, and we will slow. It is rare to find a runner over 45 who has escaped the nagging irritations from tendinitis and muscle strains.

Running causes the muscles that are active to become strong and less flexible.[7] As runners age, the loss of flexibility is exacerbated and increases the risk for injury. However, muscle mass can be at least partially maintained with strength training.

The bottom line is, while we cannot escape the aging process, there are things we can do to control how much it limits us.

How Do Social, Cultural, Emotional, and Mental Aging Factors Influence Your Running?

Of course, it is not only our bodies that change as we age. Some runners may be affected by their professional lives as they reach their most productive years, usually between their mid-forties and early sixties. These folks have less time to devote to training. Or they turn to other sports, in particular golf, for professional reasons. Networking opportunities and expectations associated with business or profession may mean spending more time with clients and associates.

For others, even if they remain interested in running, when their training partner gets a promotion or moves away, or a group run dissolves, they may lose the necessary prod to get out the door. Research shows that having a training partner is the best predictor of exercise compliance. In my role as supervisor of a physical fitness facility, I have seen dedicated runners quit or significantly reduce their adherence to training if something happens to their training partner.

Then there is the ego blow. I have seen many runners struggle mentally and emotionally with no longer being able to run as fast as they once did. I have had runners tell me that they can no longer accept running a 10-K slower than 40 minutes, or 50 minutes, or 60 minutes. Their perceptions are relative to what they could do in their prime. As a result, some reduce their serious training because they adopt an attitude of "why push myself when getting slower is inevitable."

Families can get in the way of hard training. More parents in their fifties and sixties have school-age children now than several decades ago. Even if they do not have young children, they may have grandkids or elderly parents to care for. Carving time from those kinds of responsibilities to go to the track may be hard to justify. But the more time you take away from maintaining your fitness, the harder it will be to recoup your gains as you age.

Injuries, whether running related or not, often create an interruption or a setback in training that causes a runner to become reluctant to return to vigorous training for fear of another injury. A survey of more than 500 finishers of the 1980 Peachtree Road Race (10-K) 10 years later showed that 56 percent of the entrants were still running.[8] Of those who had stopped running, 31 percent of the men and 17 percent of the women cited injury as the primary reason.

What Can Be Done? Alternatives and Solutions for the Aging Runner

What can be done to promote running as a lifelong pursuit? If entering races is a good indicator of whether runners continue to train and participate in the sport as they age, we can see that great numbers of people drop out after age 50. If you do not want to be in that group, here are some alternatives, strategies, and (hopefully) solutions for maintaining running as an appealing, enjoyable, and healthy physical activity into old age.

Runners naturally assume as that as their race times slow, their performances are not as impressive. It seems obvious. The clock ticks without mercy or judgment. That is where age grading comes in.

Some individual sports, like golf and bowling, have a method for providing a handicap so that individuals with different skill levels can be on a so-called level playing field, thus making the competition outcome uncertain. The physiological factors that affect performance as we age handicap older runners. That is why we compete in age groups, after all.

A few races, most famously the Dipsea in Northern California (the oldest trail race in the United States), use age-adjusted performances to determine race winners. That enables an 82-year-old man or a 55-year-old woman to be the race winner, even though their absolute time would not be the fastest. Some races have runners start at different times based on their age-adjusted handicaps. That allows the first person across the finish line to be the winner. This approach, in particular, creates a fun and exciting race, with the fastest runners chasing those who started much earlier based on their handicaps.

Age-adjusted tables, or an age-adjusted calculator, can be used to compare times while accounting for the vicissitudes of age. These adjustments are based on actual race times of the fastest times in the world performed by runners at every single age. Because aging is an ongoing process, being able to compare yourself with others of the exact same age provides a better snapshot of the quality of your performance.

The first age-grading tables were developed by the World Association of Veteran Athletes (WAVA), now known as World Masters Athletics (WMA).[9] WMA is the world governing body for masters track and field, long-distance running, and race walking. WAVA and *National Masters News* published those first tables in 1989. The world-record performance time for each age was computed using statistical methods rather than estimates derived from assumed rates of physiological deterioration. Revisions (taking into account improved performances at all ages) were released in 1991, 1994, 2006, 2010, and 2015.

If after applying the age adjustment to your race times, your age-adjusted graph line stays flat, you can be pleased to know that you have maintained the same performance level over time. If the age-adjusted graph line is downward, even though your actual race times may be the same or slower than times at an earlier age, the quality of your performance is higher. On the contrary, if the age-adjusted graph line moves upward, you may want to do something about your training.

My Age-Graded Performance

Below, I share a graph of my 5-K actual race times compared to my age-adjusted race times over a 35-year period; this is an example of how you can judge your race times with time adjustments made for aging. You can see that my 5-K actual race times basically stayed the same between 30 and 42, which caused the age-adjusted graph line to move downward because the expected effects of aging did not negatively affect my race times. After age 42, I got slower each year for the next 20 years. My age-adjusted race times during this 20-year period also increased. Back surgery interrupted my training for 18 months at age 45. I returned to training and marathoning but never at quite the same level of training as before. However, the rate of increase for the age-adjusted times was not as steep as that of the actual race times.

In the Preface, I described how Scott, Don, and I competed against one another when we were all much younger. In our prime,

A Comparison of 5-K Actual Race Times with Age-Adjusted Race Times for Bill Pierce, 1980-2014

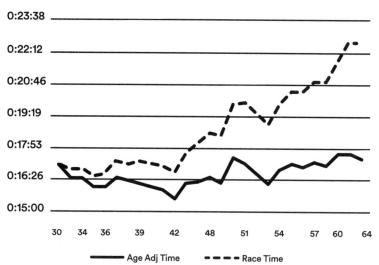

our best race times at distances from 5-K to the marathon were similar. That similarity has continued as we have aged. Our race performance times have slowed at the same rate. Because we have all three maintained the same body weight and composition and the same training regimen, aging has had an almost identical impact on our race times.

You can find age-graded standard tables and calculators for all race distances at multiple Web sites. Another metric these tables provide is a comparison of a runner's performances at different distances. That is, is your race performance at 5-K better than your half-marathon performance? Runners can compare their 5-K, 10-K, half-marathon, and full marathon race times to determine which is their best performance by using a measure called performance level percentage (PLP). See Appendix C for how PLP is computed and how it can be used to evaluate your race times at different ages.

Opportunities for Master and Senior Competitors

Many local, regional, state, and national organizations sponsor organized sports for runners ages 35 and over. Some of these focus on the highly competitive aging runner, while others hold open competitions for all aging runners with the emphasis on participation and personal gratification and development.

These organizations offer a structure for promoting interaction with other senior competitors. They give seniors a place to play. Seniors who line up to race can feel the same anxiety, excitement, and pride as when they were much younger. Participating in structured competitions provides incentive for training and a reason for setting goals. Having purpose adds vitality to your life. Many seniors find that being part of organized games reinvigorates their training.

The WMA, mentioned previously for establishing age-graded standards, was founded in 1977 to hold international championships in track and field and road racing for athletes ages 35 and over.

The USA Track & Field Association (USATF) sponsors national championships for seniors in track and field, road running, race walking, cross-country, and ultra/trail competitions. USATF state organizations also hold state senior championships in the same events.

UP CLOSE AND PERSONAL

Eve discovered running in her forties and found it empowering and freeing. She also found age-group success as she got faster and faster. That led to increased training and racing. Little attention was given to cross-training and strength training. Her 50- to 55-mile training weeks coupled with monthly long races led to a host of injuries.

Name: Eve Drinis
Age: 54
Occupation: Director of organizational development and learning
Hometown: Tampa, FL
Race times: Half-marathon, 1:45 (PR); full marathon, 3:50 (PR); recent half-marathon, 2:02
Age she began running: 40

She raced approximately 10 times per year for 12 years, including on average three or four half-marathons, one or two marathons, and one relay race. That is a lot of annual racing.

Eve's first dose of aging reality came when she realized that she could not run as much as she used to. Then she began experiencing hamstring, hip, back, and sciatica pain when she trained too aggressively or ran too much.

She knew she had to make changes in her training. She dropped her mileage from approximately 50 to 55 miles per week to 18 to 25 miles per week. She added cross-training and more strength training. As a result, she says, her core strength improved and her back issues became manageable.

The National Senior Games Association[10] sponsors the National Senior Games for athletes ages 50 and over. The Senior Games sponsors competition in 19 sports, including road race, track and field, cycling, and swimming. The State Senior Games are open to anyone 50 and over. Qualification for the National Games can be achieved at the State Games. The biennial National Senior Games attracts 12,000 competitors. State and national competitions have been held since 1985.

Every aging runner encounters those realizations eventually. What is critical is how you deal with them.

Eve's running history is a good example of how aging influences running and runners. Eve considered it a challenge to continue enjoying running and to be less focused on her race times. She says that it has proved to be an emotionally difficult task. She realizes that her slower times and more frequent injuries are a reminder that her fastest races are behind her.

She needed to reframe the training and running, she explained, not as a way to measure progress or speed but as a way to feel good, to clear her mind, to push herself without judgment. Eve embraces the idea that to train simply, to enjoy the process itself, and not to plan for any particular outcome are the keys to enjoyment.

Eve reports that her health statistics are equal to or better than a person who is in her twenties. Even though she is not getting any faster—in fact, she says that she is getting slower—she is enjoying running just as much as she used to. Like so many aging runners, she needed to get past the notion that getting slower as you age is necessarily a bad thing.

Eve's story is a familiar one. As I have pointed out throughout the book, we want to caution runners about excess and encourage more balanced training.

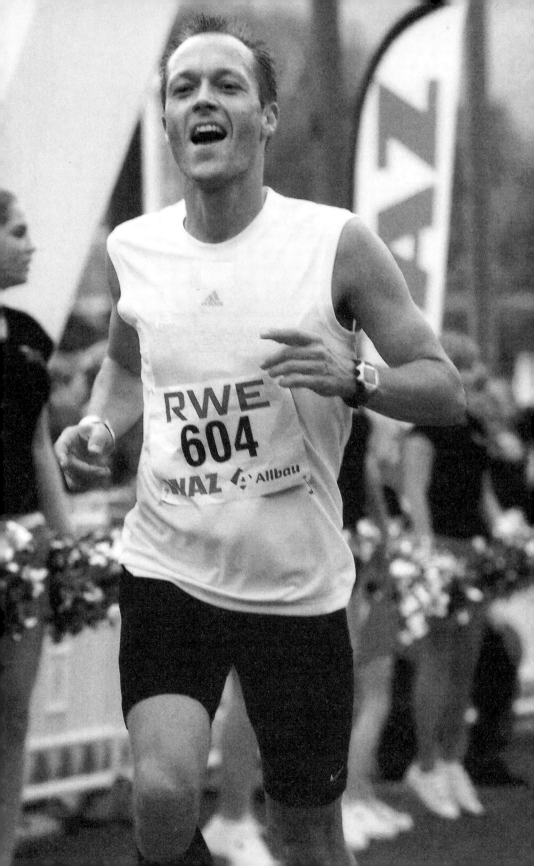

CHAPTER 3

WHY 26.2?

TWO DAYS AFTER MY 28TH BIRTHDAY, I stood on the starting line of my first marathon, having never spoken to someone who had run a marathon. Go anywhere today—supermarket, mall, movie theater—and you will spot a marathoner proudly wearing her recent race T-shirt.

In 1976, there were 25,000 marathon finishers in United States marathons. No one in 1976 could have imagined that by 2014, there would be over half a million marathon finishers in US marathons. From 300 marathons in the country in 2000 to more than 1,200 in 2014, large cities and small towns all across the country have added a marathon to expand local tourism.[1]

Why are we willing to pay hundreds of dollars to run 26.2 miles? What is responsible for the rapid growth of interest in the marathon? Why do tens of thousands of runners rush to a computer to claim an entry to a marathon race that fills all available slots in fewer than 5 minutes?

In this chapter, we explore the reasons for the marathon's appeal and rise in popularity. Even with 40 years of pleasure derived from marathons, I feel an obligation to argue that not all runners need to focus on the marathon when there is a healthier alternative.

I am going to make a modest and perhaps unpopular proposal: Instead of training for a slow marathon, I make a case for the half-marathon. The training time is less, which should reduce the overuse-injury exposure. Also, a half-marathon enables the runners to train and race at higher intensities, which will provide greater stimulations for raising their fitness levels. The half-marathon also reduces the likelihood of the long, slow finishing march, really a slow walk, commonly experienced by runners finishing in over 5 hours.

It is hard to compete with the allure of the marathon, even though half of all marathoners take $4\frac{1}{2}$ to 6 hours to finish the race. These runners are unable to store enough prerace calories to last for the whole race, so they are either left depleted or with an upset stomach from trying to ingest enough calories to supply them to the finish line. They are not racing; they are slogging through the miles. When they do their prescribed 20-milers, it is likely to take 4 or more hours. These long, slow miles do not provide the fitness benefits of higher-intensity efforts, and they increase the likelihood of overuse injuries.

Slower Runners Welcome

When I first started running marathons in the 1970s, there were marathons with 4-hour cutoffs. The marathon in San Sebastian, Spain still has a $4\frac{1}{2}$-hour finish-line cutoff.[2] Today, most marathons have at least a 6-hour finishing limit, and many are open for 8 hours to accommodate walkers. By extending the time for runners to be deemed official finishers, marathon sponsors have opened participation to a larger segment of the running population.

The median finishing time for male marathoners in 1980 was 3:32 compared with 4:19 in 2014. Median female marathon finish times were 4:03 in 1980 and 4:44 in 2014.[3]

As marathons extended the finishing cutoff times and the races attracted slower runners, there were editorials from some in the running community complaining about how slower runners were changing the sport. However, others praised the sport for opening participation to a wider cross-section of runners, for becoming more democratic and less exclusive, and for not restricting entry to only very talented runners.

For me, I support any effort to get people moving. I applaud opening races—whether it is a 5-K or a marathon—to a broader segment of the population. It has been an effective wellness initiative.

Charity Training Groups

Many charitable organizations provide a guaranteed marathon entry and 3 or 4 months of training with a coach in exchange for a charitable contribution. Some of the charity training marathons are located in attractive destinations—Disney World, Alaska, Dublin—with transportation and lodging included as part of the program. Some of these programs require the participant to raise several thousand dollars for the charity.

These programs have added to the popularity of marathoning. They have become a feature of marathons nationwide. The largest marathons all have charity programs. The Boston Marathon, as the oldest and most prestigious American marathon, has led the way with the oldest charity program and the most money raised.[4]

The Boston Marathon began a partnership with charities in 1989. Since then, hundreds of millions of dollars have been raised on behalf of charities. In 2014, an unprecedented $39.4 million was raised for charities at the Patriots' Day event. Approximately 10 percent of the runners in the 2014 event had gained entry through the reserved slots for charities.[5]

Some have complained about the entry advantage given to charity runners who are not time-qualified competitors. The complaint is that it weakens the elite status of the event.[6] I think there is room in the marathons for the charity runners. It is a way for running to contribute to the greater good of society.

Anyone who has run the Boston Marathon is familiar with the many cheers for Dana-Farber Cancer Institute charity runners. Dana-Farber has been a part of the Boston Marathon for more than 25 years, collecting $8 million from 700 runners in 2014.[7]

The Leukemia & Lymphoma Society's flagship fund-raising program is the prominent Team In Training. Since 1988, more than 600,000 participants have raised more than $1 billion for blood cancer research.[8]

There are many charity running programs, both local and national, sponsored by organizations including the Arthritis Foundation, American Stroke Association, National Parkinson Foundation, American Cancer Society, National Multiple Sclerosis Society, and Organization for Autism Research, to name a handful.

The race entries reserved for charities enable runners who wish to enter a specific marathon but did not get an entry through the lottery, or failed to enter before the race filled, to gain entry by contributing and raising money for a charity. Additionally, many runners find it inspirational to run for something bigger than themselves. Many have testified how running for a cause or to honor someone struck by a disease has enabled them to endure the training and the race distance itself. When I am running a race and I see someone whose shirt pays tribute to the memory of a loved one, it makes me think about my parents, who both were cancer victims. It is a powerful motivator.

Women Are Running, Too

The photo of Jock Semple trying to pull Kathrine Switzer off the course of the 1967 Boston Marathon has become iconic. For most young women today, it is unthinkable that they would not be allowed to run a marathon. But the fact is that in 1980, only 10 percent of all marathon finishers were female as compared with 43 percent in 2014. Marathoning prior to 1980 had been predominantly a male sport. Women were not permitted to officially run in the Boston Marathon until 1972. The growth of running and road racing, in general, has partially been fueled by the entrance of women into the sport.[9]

The passage of Title IX of the Education Amendment Act of 1972, which prevents discrimination in any education program, led to the development of high school and college sports opportunities for females. As female sports programs were slowly instituted in the 1970s and 1980s, it meant that by 1990 there was a generation of females who had participated in high school and college sports. Those women were accustomed to being physically active. Many of these women were part of the 26 percent of all marathon finishers in 1995. The 1990s saw enormous growth in the participation of young females in a wide variety of sports. These women became part of the 41 percent of all marathon finishers in 2005. That percentage slightly edged up and held for the next 10 years.[10]

In 2014, 60 percent of the Wineglass Marathon finishers in

Corning, New York, were female. Overall, women now represent 57 percent of all road race finishers.[11]

Completing a marathon feels like a huge achievement, regardless of the final time. For some, the training gives runners time to themselves, away from home, work, kids. For others, the companionship of a group provides a real sense of community and connectedness.

Bucket Lists

In recent years, many people have developed bucket lists of activities that they hope to achieve in their lifetimes. It is common to see on these lists "run a marathon" along with activities such as skydiving, visiting the Taj Mahal, reading *Don Quixote* in Spanish, hiking the Grand Canyon, and learning to play the guitar. For that reason, many marathoners enter a race for their one and only time to check off conquering the 26.2 miles.

Runners have their own running-specific bucket lists. These commonly include running a marathon in every state (50 States Marathon Club), running a marathon on all seven continents, and running in the five major marathon cities—New York, Boston, Chicago, London, and Berlin.

Races Are Big Business

While many local 5- and 10-Ks are put on as fund-raisers to buy new uniforms for the local high school marching band or raise money for a local food bank, a large number of marathons are big

business. Race directors focus on expanding the number of participants to increase the race revenue. By adding shorter race
options—5-K, 10-K, half-marathon, and a marathon relay—to a
marathon, the race event can increase its total participation by 3 to
10 times. Also, by leaving the race course open longer, the race will
attract walkers and slower runners, which adds significantly to the
entry-fee revenues.

The entry fee for the New York City Marathon in 1970 was $1.[12]
In 2015, that same NYC Marathon entry was $255 for US residents
and $357 for international runners. With more than 50,000 people
entered in the race, we're talking big bucks.

The Rock 'n' Roll Marathon Series, which conducted its first
marathon in San Diego in 2000, sponsors 30 events in the United
States, Canada, Mexico, and Ireland, with more than 600,000 runners participating.[13] When the race is a celebration, with bands and
a party atmosphere in a destination city, it can draw runners from
around the world.

Other companies and nonprofit organizations recognize how
lucrative it can be to conduct an event for tens of thousands of runners. Local cities are eager to partner with race sponsors to draw
thousands of visitors for multiday stays. The impact on local econ-
omies is significant.

Road races are attractive to sponsors. That is why the back of
your race T-shirt is covered with corporate logos. Sponsorships for
most races are available at multiple levels. For some of the larger
marathons, title sponsorships are multiple-year deals worth millions of dollars. Lower-level sponsorships may involve in-kind services or products. Sports drinks, financial services, luxury
automobiles, and shoe companies are often lead sponsors. These
sponsors are eager to generate name recognition among the

thousands of participants who fit their consumers' financial pro-files. When multiple sponsors underwrite a large portion of event expenses, the race can be quite profitable.

Race companies recognize the opportunities for growing their businesses and brands and have expanded into international ven-ues. Marathoning in Asia has exploded, with hundreds of races established in the 21st century.

Sharing the Experience

Many runners have become marathoners as a result of a "let's run a marathon" conversation among friends. "I'll do it if you will" can lead to selecting a race, often at an attractive destination, and the need to develop a training plan. Then comes making travel and lodging reservations and beginning the special bonding that devel-ops from training together to meet the challenge. The experience becomes much more about the shared training runs, heartfelt training-run conversations, elation over good training runs, despondency associated with bad runs and injuries, and the cama-raderie developed over several months than about the race itself.

I have run 42 marathons, 26 of them with my brother. We have trained and raced together for more than 40 years. Our race times are nearly identical, and we never know which of us is going to cross the finish line first. We usually run side by side until one of us pulls away near the end. In races of all distances, our winning percentage against each other is right at 50 percent. We truly race with each other as much as we race against each other. We develop our strategy together and help pace each other in races. However, we also try to push each other. It is ideal to have a running partner

UP CLOSE AND PERSONAL

W e all have a lot to learn from Jim. At 46, he began jogging to lose weight and get healthier. He reports that at age 50, he still needed to lose 35 more pounds to be at his high school weight. He targeted running a marathon to give him that extra incentive for reaching his ideal weight. He did that the next year and has maintained his weight and marathoning for a little over 25 years.

Name: Jim Michie
Age: 78
Occupation: Real estate
Hometown: Salt Lake City, UT
Race times: Marathon, 3:00
Age he began running: 46

Jim qualified for and ran the Boston Marathon at age 53. Eighty-year-old John Kelly was in the race that year. He had won the Boston Marathon twice and finished it 58 times. Jim decided then that his goal was to run the Boston Marathon at age 80.

Jim made marathoning his hobby. He has completed 59 marathons in destinations all across the country. He enjoys the travel and invites family members to join him to run or observe. He is delighted that he has been able to inspire his daughters and sons-in-law to run and choose healthy lifestyles.

What is most inspiring about Jim's running is that he takes no prescription medications, and all of his health indices from his annual physical exams are excellent. Not many in their late seventies can report the same.

Jim's age-adjusted marathon time at age 75 was a 2:50. His training is not only contributing to his good health but is also keeping him fast.

Jim runs 3 days per week and cross-trains on his nonrunning days. He goes to the gym regularly and does strength training to maintain his muscle mass. He reports that stretching contributes to his ability to keep running.

Jim knows that I would prefer that he run fewer marathons each year, but it is his hobby. He enjoys the travel and the healthy family involvement. Maybe I can convince him that substituting a few half-marathons in the next 2 years will increase the likelihood of his being able to toe the line at Hopkinton at age 80.

who pulls you along with encouragement until the finish line is in sight—and then it is every man for himself.

Of course, I am doubly blessed with good training partners. My coauthor, Scott Murr, and I have shared 4,000 training runs together. Training partners develop deep friendships, one of the benefits of running. For those not lucky enough to have colleagues or friends for training partners, running clubs provide motivation for consistent training and a social outlet.

Experiencing Special Destinations

In a marathon, you can tour the monuments of Washington, DC, run through all five boroughs of New York City, or traverse the city of Chicago by running up the middle of LaSalle Street. These truly special experiences attract thousands of runners.

I choose marathons for their unique courses and scenery. Some of my favorites have been in the western states of Arizona, Colorado, Idaho, Nevada, Utah, and Washington. The reliably cool, dry mornings make that region of the country attractive for marathoning, even though performances can suffer with the effects of altitude and, sometimes, strong winds. The spectacular scenery makes the races breathtaking in more ways than one.

Now many small towns sponsor marathons. The locals embrace the events and are proud to showcase their towns to out-of-state runners. They treat all runners as special guests. I consider my experiences in places like Ashton, Idaho; Ashland, Wisconsin; and Bemidji, Minnesota, every bit as special as running in Boston, New York, and Chicago.

A couple of international running opportunities provided me with special cultural experiences. The Usedom Marathon starts in

Swinoujscie, Poland, and finishes in Wolgast, Germany. Running with Poles, Russians, and Germans and postrace interactions with locals made the marathon a memorable experience. Sharing the challenge of 26.2 miles creates a bond that overcomes the barrier of language.

The Mystery

Sports fans are attracted to uncertain outcomes. We get excited about close games. We take care not to learn the results of delayed broadcast events. How many of us turn off the news when the Olympics are in an earlier time zone?

Runners generally know within a few seconds what their 5-K or 10-K race times will be. Even half-marathon performances are fairly predictable. That is where the marathon differs. Each marathon is a mystery that unfolds over 26.2 miles. Most marathoners never know how they will hold up after 20 miles.

The choice of a too-fast early pace, a misjudgment of the effects of race-day heat and humidity, a race-week cold or sinus infection, or a bad dietary selection the day before or morning of the race can undermine 16-plus weeks of preparation and result in a miserable, slow march to the finish line. Sometimes everything seems perfect and the poor performance is inexplicable.

It is this uncertainty that keeps many runners returning to the marathon for that optimal performance. Because there are few opportunities to run a great marathon—ideal weather combined with excellent training—marathoners come back to the roads for that race where all the elements come together for the performance that meets their dream expectations. And when it happens, the finish line becomes drowned in emotion.

The Joy of the Journey

I tell people that if they want to run a marathon, they have to enjoy the journey. The race itself lasts only a few hours, but the preparation is spread over several months. The enjoyment that I get from focused training for 4 months leads me to submit a marathon entry year after year. I like to use a 16-week marathon-training schedule. The weekend long runs, and seeing how I get stronger week after week as the long runs move from 10 to 20 miles, sustain me through the related fatigue. Having a goal I can visualize during those 16 weeks keeps me focused on training as well as the excitement of anticipation—and a little trepidation—as the race draws near.

But Is It Healthy?

Most serious marathoners train for reasons other than good health. The psychosocial reinforcement associated with performance and achievement can be a powerful motivator.

As marathoning continues to gain popularity throughout the world, will it contribute not only to the high rate of injuries associated with marathon training but also to potential long-term, harmful health consequences for those who pursue the sport over many years? Is there a threshold where the amount of training crosses from healthy to harmful? Does that threshold vary for individuals?

Marathons require a weekly long run that often leaves runners fatigued to the point where they cannot play ball with their kids or clean the bathroom. Many marathoners are eager to get to the race so that they can end the stress of the weekly long training run; many of their families are equally eager for them to reach the end of the training commitment and resume their regular life.

Marathon training can lead to bad postural habits from running lots of slow miles. The physical stress from higher mileage can contribute to a weakened immune system and increased vulnerability to colds, flu, and other respiratory ailments. The additional time spent running and the concomitant fatigue often mean less time and energy for performing important resistance training and stretching.

Is there a healthier alternative? Runners, coaches, and researchers have identified the half-marathon as a way to enjoy the benefits thought to accrue to marathoners but without all the risks associated with the full distance of 26.2 miles.

The Healthier Alternative

A growing number of runners have come to see the half-marathon as the perfect race distance. It provides the challenges and benefits of the marathon with fewer of its disadvantages. Half-marathons require focused training, but the big difference is that the typical long training run is 10 miles, in contrast to the marathon long training run of 20 miles. Recovery from a 10-mile training run is much easier than from a training run of twice that distance.

For most runners, with proper training the half-marathon can be raced. Running hard for 2 hours or slightly more is within the capability of trained runners. Think about it. That is how long elite runners race in the marathon. The average marathon runner is running for 4 hours or more, which makes the event one of enduring and surviving rather than racing.

More destination races are offering half-marathons along with marathons, though runners at these events often hang their heads when asked which distance they are running. They can feel somehow inadequate if they are only running half. Rachel Toor, *Running Times* columnist and author of *Personal Record,* called for a new half-marathon name—the Thirteener.[14] She added, "It's not half of something; it's a whole thing."

Fortunately, the half-marathon is enjoying immense popularity, thanks to the perhaps wiser runners. There were more than 2,200 US half-marathon races in 2014.[15]

In 2014, the half-marathon distance surpassed 2 million finishers in the United States, and females composed 61 percent of the finishers. According to Running USA's 2015 National Runner Survey, the half-marathon distance is the favorite race distance of runners nationwide.[16]

Perhaps more runners will realize that the half-marathon may be the healthier alternative and, as Toor explained, a half is the whole thing.

CHAPTER 4

IS LONG-DISTANCE RUNNING HEALTHY?

IT SEEMS THAT EVERY TIME you read the news, you encounter a report on the latest research examining the effects of running on heart health. Marathon deaths always receive a lot of attention in the press. That is because marathoning is perceived as an extreme activity.

In truth, anytime you get 40,000 people together to engage in a taxing physical activity, it is likely that someone's going to have a bad day. Research about sudden deaths in marathons indicates that there are approximately 0.75 deaths per 100,000 marathon race participants.[1] As the number of participants increases, the number of sudden deaths increases. Most autopsies show that the deaths were related to preexisting cardiovascular disease and not linked to physical conditioning.

As a graduate student in the mid-1970s, I read an article that quoted Thomas Bassler, MD, a California pathologist, who proclaimed that marathon running would prevent fatty deposits in the blood.[2] He further stated boldly that anyone who ran a marathon under 4 hours was protected against coronary heart disease. It was this promise of heart disease immunity, along with my family history of heart disease, that caused me to switch my primary activity from basketball to distance running.

Recently, the major newspapers grabbed the attention of runners with headlines reporting the results of a 2012 study by James H. O'Keefe, MD, a research cardiologist. He and his coauthors report that while regular exercise was effective in promoting cardiovascular health and preventing chronic diseases, long-term excessive exercise may lead to pathological restructuring of the heart and large arteries. He concludes that there is evidence that long-term excessive, sustained exercise may be associated with coronary artery calcification, diastolic dysfunction, and large-artery wall stiffening.[3]

Anyone who is reading this book knows that exercise is a good thing. But what is the right amount?

The 2008 report of the Centers for Disease Control and Prevention's Physical Activity Advisory Committee recommended 150 minutes per week of moderate-intensity or 75 minutes per week of vigorous-intensity aerobic exercise for all US adults.[4] According to the Council on Clinical Cardiology, regular physical activity reduces cardiovascular disease and death.[5]

Most Americans do not meet these recommendations. We seem to be a country of extremes—either no exercise or lots of exercise. All of us need to find the right balance.

Because these recommendations have been widely recognized and adopted, the recent and surprising reports suggesting that high volumes of aerobic exercise may be bad for cardiovascular health have drawn much attention. Most runners easily exceed the recommendations for the number of weekly minutes of vigorous intensity.

Often runners are left to trial and error to determine those thresholds of what is beneficial and what is harmful. And how about individual differences? Sport scientists know the amount of exercise to achieve optimal fitness varies among individuals. Maybe health benefit thresholds, like training thresholds, also vary by individual. But can there be too much of a good thing?

Let us begin by taking a quick look at how what is commonly called the exercise boom began. Prior to 1970, it was unusual to see a fitness center or hear public health messages that encouraged regular exercise. What have been the consequences of the emphasis on the importance of exercise for good health? Are there unintended consequences associated with the increased emphasis and the desire to go beyond the recommended levels of aerobic activity?

What Fueled America's Exercise and Running Boom?

One man gets a lot of the credit for getting Americans to move. Many consider the publication of Kenneth Cooper, MD's *Aerobics*, which has sold more than 2 million copies, as a major factor in drawing the public's attention to the benefits of physical activity. While in the US Air Force, Dr. Cooper developed the 12-minute run to assess fitness, and after he left the service, he opened the Cooper Clinic in Dallas in 1970.

In Dr. Cooper's landmark book, he laid out a point system to keep track of fitness. It was in this book that he introduced the term "aerobics," which became a common term for physical activity demanding an increased consumption of oxygen. Since 1970, the Cooper Clinic has produced countless research studies to confirm his 1968 hypothesis that cardiorespiratory fitness is related to improved health and longevity.

Dr. Bassler's bold promise about the prevention of heart disease (even if exaggerated for attention) influenced me as a graduate student and many others. He contributed to the growing interest and participation in road racing. And so 10-K races sprung up in communities all across the country. He helped found the Honolulu Marathon. He even trained several heart attack patients to run the Honolulu Marathon to emphasize the value of exercise as part of cardiac rehabilitation.[6]

Dr. Bassler's influence helped promote road racing participation. He created enthusiasm for the health benefits associated with distance running. Then in 1984, the death of popular author and runner Jim Fixx quelled some of the optimism created by Dr. Bassler. Fixx, author of the million-copy best seller *The Complete Book of Running,* died at age 42 while on a run. This provided cynics with loads of ammunition to shoot down the idea that jogging was healthy and safe for older adults.

The major running magazines ran articles explaining that Fixx's father had a heart attack at age 35 and died 8 years later. An autopsy showed that Fixx had an 80 percent blockage of a coronary artery.[7] Fixx not only had a family history of heart disease, he was also overweight and a longtime smoker before he began running.

Dr. Cooper played a major role in alleviating runners' anxieties over Fixx's death. In response, he wrote *Running Without Fear,* a book that explained the role of heredity, coupled with years of poor health habits, as a contributor to Fixx's untimely death. Dr. Cooper wanted the public to know that running had most likely prolonged Fixx's life rather than caused his death. However, we should not be surprised to see continuing articles that question the safety of running and vigorous exercise each time a death occurs in a running or endurance event.

In 1997, approximately 30 years after the publication of

Aerobics, Dr. Cooper expressed concern about very frequent high-intensity exercise.

Studies from his clinic showed that regular exercisers lived longer compared to those who were sedentary—with the exception of those who exercised the most. He cited a list of well-known devoted runners, cyclists, and triathletes who had encountered cancer and heart disease. Dr. Cooper attributed the contraction of these ailments to free radicals, the unstable oxygen molecules identified as contributing to chronic diseases. He concluded that if your exercise exceeds running more than 15 miles per week, or its equivalent, you are doing it for a reason other than health.[8]

A number of experts recommend moderation. John Mandrola, MD, a cardiac electrophysiologist and competitive cyclist, wrote: "Exercise is the best therapeutic intervention a doctor has to offer. It's safe, it's effective, and, yes, it's beautiful. But like everything else in life, too much of a good thing can lead to trouble. What we don't know is how much is too much. Dosing exercise seems similar to dosing medicine: One patient's high dose is another's toxic dose."[9] As with training, individuals have different thresholds for tolerating stress and different reactions to the inflammation from that stress.

Dr. O'Keefe advocates moderation. He cites evidence that no exercise or too little exercise has no health benefits, and that too much—more than 25 miles per week—can be harmful.[10] He cautions against extreme endurance exercise over many years and decades.

Findings from recent British,[11] Danish,[12] and German[13] studies have indicated that strenuous running raises the risk of cardiovascular disease. However, because of the cited limitations of these studies, it is premature to conclude that high volumes of exercise increase cardiovascular disease.

The Benefits of Cardiorespiratory Fitness

Any physical activity that gets your heart rate up and keeps it up for a prolonged period of time will benefit your cardiorespiratory fitness. For optimal results, you should have an exercise plan that details mode, intensity, duration, and frequency.

The benefits of a well-rounded fitness program have been confirmed in numerous studies over the past 50 years. Some of the benefits that have been identified include:

- Lowered risk of cardiovascular disease
- Increased VO_2 max
- Increased muscular endurance
- Increased immune function
- Increased number of capillaries
- Increased number of mitochondria in muscle cells
- Increased bone density
- Reduced body fat
- Reduced cholesterol levels
- Increased high-density lipoproteins (HDL)
- Reduced risk of type 2 diabetes
- Reduced risk of certain types of cancer
- Increased self-esteem
- Improved sleep
- Reduced fatigue
- Increased longevity

If you are reading this book, you probably do not need to be convinced of the health benefits of exercise. The science is on your side.

Ralph S. Paffenbarger Jr., MD, a surgeon and epidemiologist whose landmark study substantiated the link between exercise and longevity, helped lay the foundation for the modern fitness movement. His landmark College Alumni Health Study investigated the exercise habits of more than 50,000 University of Pennsylvania and Harvard University alumni. The study confirmed that more physically active people have a lower risk of coronary heart disease. He found that death rates declined steadily as energy expended on physical activity increased from less than 500 calories of energy expended per week to 2,000 or more calories of energy expended in physical activity per week.[14]

Paul T. Williams, PhD, at the Department of Energy's Lawrence Berkeley National Laboratory has conducted the National Runners' and Walkers' Health Study since the 1990s. The study has produced more than 65 peer-reviewed articles over 20 years that show lower rates of disease in runners and walkers. The study has followed 113,472 runners and 42,012 walkers on their exercise habits and health histories.[15]

The cohorts currently include more than 150,000 subjects, which also makes them among the largest epidemiological cohorts in the world. This research shows that exercise is associated with:

❱ 40% lower brain cancer risk

❱ 76% lower kidney cancer risk

❱ 41% lower breast cancer mortality

❱ 37% lower pneumonia mortality

❱ 45% lower sepsis mortality

❱ 45% lower risk for hip replacement

❱ 42% lower risk for cataracts

❱ 32% lower incidence of cardiac arrhythmias

- 40% lower risk for chronic kidney disease per mile/day run in hypertensives
- 33% lower risk for benign prostate hyperplasia
- 52% lower risk for gallbladder disease

UP CLOSE AND PERSONAL

John is an active member of the Florida Track Club in Gainesville. He enjoys the camaraderie with club members who often socialize after workouts. He is a good example of someone who in midlife rediscovered the social and health benefits of running.

Name: John Davis

Age: 56

Occupation: Professor of forest biotechnology and molecular biology

Hometown: Gainesville, FL

Race times: Most recent and best-ever marathon, 3:15; most recent and best-ever 5-K, 19:43

Age he began running: Mid-40s

John began training more seriously with his fellow club members and ran his fastest marathon at age 55. His BMI of 21.8, 10 percent body fat, and overall healthy dietary habits certainly enabled him to have success at a time when most runners begin to slow.

It is perplexing to try to understand why 7 months after John's eighth and fastest marathon, during a phase of slow, easy running, he had a heart attack. He was fit and thin. We like to think that a combination of good diet and exercise prevents heart disease. That was not true for John.

John was unlucky to have a heart attack, but he was lucky where it happened. John experienced the heart attack while on vacation in Seattle just after an easy run. He was immediately taken to a state-of-the-art facility and given immediate treatment and a stent. His rehab and recovery started immediately.

Even a fast marathoner with a healthy diet and low body fat is not protected from a heart attack. John's case is a sobering reminder of our vulnerability. Fortunately, John received excellent emergency care.

- 45% lower risk for gout

- 48% lower risk for diverticular disease

- 54% lower risk for macular degeneration

- 43% lower risk for glaucoma[16]

Epidemiologists have identified a family history of heart disease, high blood sugar, high blood pressure, smoking, obesity, a sedentary lifestyle, poor diet, and high cholesterol as coronary risk factors. John had none of these risks except for high cholesterol. While his total cholesterol level was elevated (220), his HDLs—the good cholesterol—were very high (85), making his total cholesterol to HDL ratio very low. One's cholesterol ratio is considered a better risk predictor for heart disease than total cholesterol. The lower the ratio, the lower the risk.

Because of his low risk for heart disease as determined by the low cholesterol ratio, John chose not to take a statin drug, even though he and his physician had an ongoing discussion as to whether he should be taking one. Now he takes one daily.

One factor potentially related to John's unfortunate cardiac event is that for 4 weeks prior to his heart attack, he took a high daily dose of a prescribed nonsteroidal anti-inflammatory drug (NSAID) to relieve pain from a rotator cuff injury. Interestingly, a few days before his attack, the FDA strengthened its warning linking nonaspirin NSAID use and heart attacks—even in patients with no history of cardiovascular disease.

It bears repeating that one is never immune from coronary heart disease regardless of diet, exercise, and medication.

John's positive attitude and cardiac rehabilitation enabled him to return to the activity that he enjoys. His high level of fitness from running may have contributed to his survival and his recovery.

Whenever a devoted marathoner experiences a heart attack, questions are raised as to whether the physical stress of excessive effort contributed to the attack. We hope the discussion in this chapter provides an understanding of the cardiac health benefits of endurance training, as well as the concerns of cardiac researchers about the potential risks.

What Can We Conclude from These Studies?

We all want our exercise to be beneficial without doing any harm to our long-term health. However, many serious runners are similar to competitive athletes in other sports who are willing to assume the risks associated with their sports. We cannot ignore the research studies of the past 10 years. For those of us who have trained continuously and vigorously over multiple decades, there is naturally concern as to whether our exercise regimens will provide the optimal health and longevity we were targeting. For those much younger, the recent research findings provide a reason to pay close attention to the latest science to determine the ideal dose of running for optimal health.

For the past few years, FIRST has had the good fortune of having Michael S. Emery, MD, and fellow of the American College of Cardiology, participate in our retreats. He has had considerable experience with runners and their heart health. Dr. Emery was one of the volunteer physicians in the medical tent at the 2013 Boston Marathon, only 100 yards away from the terrorist explosion. He is the medical director of the IU Health Center for Cardiovascular Care in Athletics at the Indiana University School of Medicine.

Because of his serious interest in running and sports coupled with his expertise in sports cardiology, I asked Dr. Emery to help interpret the recent research claiming that excessive endurance training may have deleterious consequences for health. We discussed the research reported in a 2016 article that Dr. Emery coauthored. Here are some of the findings and conclusions from that article, "Exercise at the Extremes: The Amount of Exercise to Reduce Cardiovascular Events," published in the *Journal of the American College of Cardiology*.[17]

- Recreational marathon training has been shown to have a positive effect on cardiovascular risk.

- Lifelong patterns of "committed" exercise and "competitive" masters-level athletes prevent many cardiovascular disorders.

- Runners have lower all-cause and cardiovascular death rates.

- Athletes performing the highest exercise volumes do not demonstrate any increased risk for cardiovascular disease. The possibility that too much exercise training could produce harmful cardiac effects is worthy of further scientific investigation.

- There may be individuals with genetic predispositions for cardiac disease for whom exercise training is not beneficial.

- Overall, a very active, lifelong participation in exercise training outweighs any risks.

For now, at least, I do not see any reason to put our running shoes on the shelf. Although for me, I am going to focus on 5-Ks to half-marathons, primarily because the training for them is more manageable and enjoyable. As always, we should pay attention to our bodies and not ignore symptoms of concern and signs of change that cannot be easily explained.

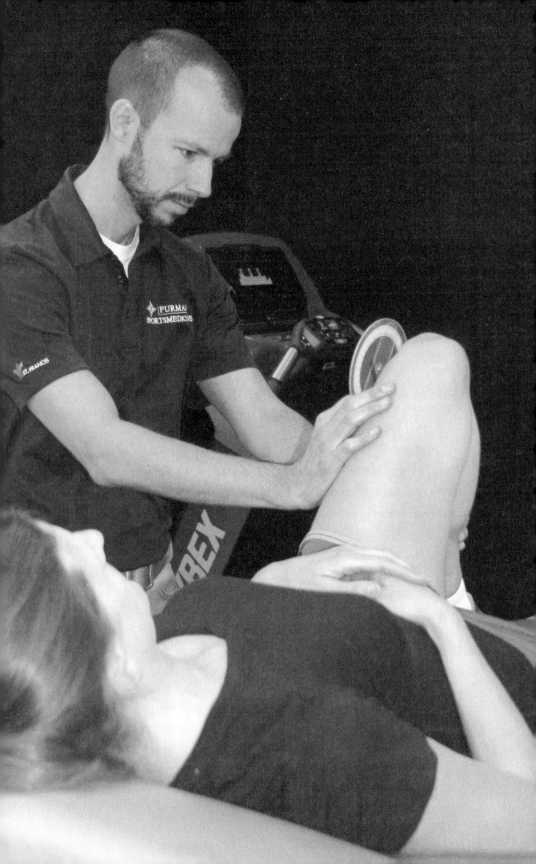

CHAPTER 5

WHY DO I GET INJURED WHEN I AM SO SINCERE?

WHILE MARATHONING CAN BE EXPENSIVE and time-consuming, running is perhaps the most egalitarian physical activity. Nearly everyone can do it. You can run by yourself or with others, in all kinds of weather, on all kinds of terrain, at all times of the day or night, with minimal equipment costs. And running requires virtually no skill to get started.

The drawback to running often comes down to a single issue: injuries. The estimates for the percentage of runners who will sustain an overuse injury in a given year vary from 40 to 80 percent. Even when minor in nature, injuries are always frustrating and at times can become serious.

There's a *Peanuts* cartoon I love where Charlie Brown asks, "How do we lose when we're so sincere?" Runners share a similar sentiment. Runners are dedicated, disciplined, determined, and faithful to the plan. Maybe their sincerity is a source of injuries because they are unwilling to interrupt their training.

Identifying the source of an injury is often a challenge. In most cases, the injury is a result of multiple factors. There are hundreds of studies searching for the primary causes of running injuries. The confounding results typically have focused on anatomical structures, training volume, type of training, running form, types of shoes, muscular strength, flexibility, psychological issues, and previous injury history as potential causes of injuries.

At FIRST, we receive many messages from runners asking for advice on how to treat an injury. Runners want to know why they got injured, how the injury should be treated, whether they should stop running, or if they have had to stop running, what they need to do to resume their running and when they can resume.

The best predictor of an individual's developing an injury is having had a previous injury. So don't get injured! Injury prevention is of utmost importance. A little prehab planning can prevent post-injury rehab. That is why we developed the 7-Hour Workout Week.

Runners often get injured when they prepare for a race—in particular, for a marathon. Because they have already invested a lot of effort, time, and emotional energy in their preparation, they are reluctant to stop running at the first signs of an injury. They think, *I'll just keep running for a few more weeks, and then after the race, I'll rest and recover.* This attitude generally leads to a more serious injury. Had the runners responded immediately and altered their racing plans and goals until the injury was treated, they could have been back on track to recover much more quickly.

Most runners, like teenagers, want to believe in their own invincibility and neglect precautionary advice. Runners in general are able to run without concern for injury for a lengthy period of time, sometimes years, before the cumulative stress of repetitive impact results in an injury. This particularly applies to younger runners. Bad habits, which may not have initially contributed to an injury but that lead to problems later, are hard to break.

FIRST has been very fortunate to have D. S. Blaise Williams III, PhD, MPT, director of the VCU RUN LAB and associate professor of physical therapy at Virginia Commonwealth University, as part of its retreat faculty. Dr. Williams, a biomechanist and physical therapist, is an acknowledged expert in gait analysis and running injury treatment.

He provides every participant of the FIRST retreats with an individualized gait analysis. He takes measurements of participants' lower limbs to look for any differences between the left and right legs, examines arches of the feet, and measures range of motion to unearth flexibility issues. He carefully analyzes their treadmill running video and marks mechanical flaws. He then advises retreat participants on the stretches and strengthening exercises that they need to do, as well as the postural changes they should practice.

Many runners attend our retreats seeking a solution for an injury that limits or prevents their training. Dr. Williams has many admirers who are grateful for his accurate diagnoses and detailed rehabilitation plans that have enabled them to return to vigorous training and racing.

Here you will find Dr. Williams's responses to the most common running injury questions that we receive.

Q. There are training programs that call for anywhere from 3 to 7 days per week of running. Is there a relationship between frequency of running and running-related injury?

A. The short answer for most runners is: Less is more. Studies published in each decade over the last 30 years agree that the most common factor related to injuries is weekly mileage and days per week running.[1] One study found that running 30 minutes per day for 3 days per week resulted in an injury rate of 12 to 24 percent, while running 5 days per week for 30 minutes resulted in an injury rate of 39 percent. Furthermore, those who ran 5 days per week for 45 minutes had an injury rate of 54 percent.[2]

How often should you run? This is an interesting question that likely varies for everyone. Advocates for daily running and high mileage suggest neuromuscular changes and cardiovascular changes necessary for high-level performance can only occur with high-mileage training.

While some individuals can run daily without detrimental effects, most individuals cannot maintain such a heavy training load. Over the last 2 years, we have completed a series of studies through the VCU RUN LAB with individuals who were training for a half-marathon. As part of this study, we compared 3-day- versus 5-day-per-week training programs. The results from this study demonstrated that training 5 days per week did not result in increased performance during training or on race day.

In addition, daily questionnaires revealed that runners were happiest when they ran more than 3 days per week and fewer than 5 days per week with 1 day of cross-training (nonrunning). Based on these results, we recommend running 3 or 4 days per week. This is nice, because it allows for running every other day with 1 or 2 cross-training days per week and 2 or 3 days off per week. This allows for adequate variability of exercise and opportunity for musculoskeletal recovery.

Q. Is there a weekly mileage threshold that increases the likelihood of injury?

A. While there is no fixed mileage, there are reports that suggest that more than 20 miles per week increases the likelihood of injury.[3] Studies show that the relative risk of injury is significantly greater (two to three times) when running 40 or more miles per week.[4]

Of course, your weekly mileage will change depending on the race distance you are training for. For example, marathon trainers will have long runs of 20 miles throughout their training. These weeks are likely to approach a minimum of 30 to 35 miles of total running. The key is to reduce your miles the next week so that the *average* mileage over your 16- to 20-week program approaches 25 to 30 miles. If you are training for a 10-K or half-marathon, it is much easier to keep your mileage threshold down. The bottom line is: You need to establish where your weekly mileage threshold is and adjust your weekly training to stay at or below that mileage. Unfortunately, this usually is accomplished by trial and error. However, finding the threshold will keep your legs happy and allow adequate recovery time.

Q. Does running fast lead to injury?

A. There are no explicit data that suggest that running fast leads to injury. However, running fast does require that the muscles work harder and at faster angular velocities. In order for this to occur, the muscles need to transfer between concentric and eccentric muscle activity more effectively. If a runner is not accustomed to running fast, these efforts could increase the risk of injury. Most people couldn't bench press 300 pounds on their first try; it takes practice and training. The same is true for running fast; steadily increase your exposure to running fast and you'll likely stay healthy.

Q. Is body weight related to the risk of running-related injury?

A. There are conflicting results on this factor. Some studies say yes.[5] Others say no.[6] So now you're thinking, "Great, I don't have to lose weight" or "My weight isn't related to my injury." The fact is, with every pound we gain, we add 3 to 4 pounds of weight with every step. This also adds 10 to 15 pounds of pressure per step to our knee and hip joints. While this may not directly relate to injury, it surely places quite a bit of demand and stress on the muscles and cartilage. It's best to try to maintain a healthy weight to minimize your risk of injury. Not to mention the fact that carrying extra weight slows down performance.

Q. Is heel-striking bad? Is it inefficient or will it cause me to run slowly? Does it lead to injury?

A. This is a great question that has received much attention in recent years. Technically, there is a difference between "heel-striking" and "rear-foot striking." Heel-striking is characterized by a long stride to the front with toes pointed toward the sky and is associated with high impacts at initial contact.

Very few runners actually heel-strike. Most long-distance runners (approximately 90 percent) are rear-foot strikers.[7] Rear-foot striking is characterized by landing on the rear end of the foot at initial contact. The impact on the body for rear-foot strikers is not as forceful as it is for heel-strikers. Rear-foot striking is no less efficient than midfoot- or forefoot-striking as long as the same stride rate is maintained.[8]

When a runner's foot makes contact with the ground, the body must absorb that force. Rear-foot strikers absorb most of the force with their knees, while midfoot-strikers absorb the force in their arches and calves. The reason that runners with heel-strike patterns versus mid/forefoot-strike patterns get different injuries is because they absorb force in different areas.

Most biomechanical running studies conclude that there is no one best footstrike pattern. Many lower-leg injuries are a result of over-striding rather than footstrike patterns. In general, if you sustain an injury, having a gait analysis or knowledgeable running coach determine if you overstride may be your first step before you try changing your footstrike pattern.

Q. Does running form contribute to injuries? How do I know if my running form is okay?

A. As a running biomechanist, it would be blasphemy for me to say that running form does not contribute to injury. However, it is not the only factor related to injury and is certainly controversial in the literature. There are some factors that are more convincing than others when it comes to running form. Specifically, hip control[9] and stride rate[10] seem to be most convincing.

The most practical way to decide if your form is okay is to assess your health and performance. If you can continue to train and improve your performance while staying injury-free, you are likely to have reasonable running form. A running analysis performed by a trained professional can provide you with valuable information regarding your running form and efficiency.

Q. Is changing running form recommended? Should runners try to change their running form or try to improve their own natural running form?

A. For most healthy runners, changing running form is not needed. There are no data to suggest that changing from one form to another will improve your performance or reduce your risk of injury. However, if you are injured, changing running form may be an option to reduce or eliminate your symptoms. The easiest way to change your running form is to increase your stride rate.

Changing stride rate can be fun and add variety to your training week. First, you need to know your stride rate. This is best done at your comfortable training pace and can be accomplished by counting your steps over 30 seconds or a minute. If you are below 160 steps per minute, you are on the low side and could likely benefit from an increase.

Data suggest that changes of 5 to 7 percent in stride rate are easily obtained and maintained. Anything more than this is too much. For example, if you have knee pain and your step rate is 150 steps per minute, you can increase to 158 to 160 steps per minute in a single session. This is best done on a treadmill with a free metronome app. Practice for about 2 or 3 weeks, and it should become natural.

Q. Does running contribute to arthritis and/or the likelihood of a need for future knee and hip replacements?

A. Absolutely not. In fact, long-term studies prove otherwise. Individuals who participated in running for physical activity at any time during their life were more likely to live longer and less likely to develop diseases and pathologies, including arthritis. While there are no specific data on running and total joint replacements, there is little need for total joint replacements without the presence of advanced osteoarthritis.[11]

Q. What are the primary causes of hip pain?

A. Hip pain, like all other lower-extremity pain, can come from many sources. Muscle soreness after runs is common around the hip, and as long as this resolves within 1 or 2 days, it is probably nothing to worry about. Pain that is persistent or increases in intensity or duration during and after your runs is likely more serious. Hip pain can be related to muscle strains of the hip flexors, abductors, or extensors (glutes and hamstrings). Deeper pain may be more serious and related to changes in the joint surface or to the cartilage of the hip. Changes in strength, flexibility, and motor control may be contributing factors to all types of hip pain.

Q. How do I prevent a hamstring injury?

A. While there is no definite way to prevent running injuries, there are known factors that may benefit the runner in maintaining strong and efficient muscles. The hamstrings are primarily responsible for slowing the leg down just before foot contact. Both flexibility[12] and strength[13] of the hamstrings are important factors in maintaining their health. Dynamic flexibility exercises and functional strengthening exercises can be beneficial in maintaining the health of the hamstrings. (See the exercises in Chapter 13.)

Q. Is there any relationship between running injuries and stretching? Do you recommend stretching?

A. There is some evidence to suggest that individuals who stretch on an inconsistent basis may be more likely to get injured. In particular, asymmetry of flexibility seems to be the greatest predictor of injury. Therefore, if one hamstring or calf is less flexible than the other, it may be beneficial to even them out. There do not appear to be any detrimental effects of stretching, and stretching can often make runners feel "looser" before a run or help them cool down after a run.

A couple rules of thumb: Don't stretch cold, and don't aggressively stretch, particularly after a long run. In all of these situations, the runner is more likely to stretch the muscle beyond its physiological limits and result in a microtear or strain. Remember, stretching is intended to help the muscle prepare for activity or recover. It should never cause pain during or after.

Q. How important is strength training for injury avoidance? Do you recommend strength training?

A. Most runners develop weakness in certain muscles over time. This can be related to poor form, lack of cross-training, or muscle imbalances related to flexibility or previous injuries. Common areas for muscle weakness in runners are hip abductors, hip external rotators, hamstrings, and calves. Runners can benefit from strength training, but the training needs to extend outside the fitness machines. Functional strengthening of the lower extremities leading to exercises for neuromuscular control such as lunges and squats is necessary to transfer the strength to the unique demands of running. (See the exercises in Chapter 12.)

In general, research data do not suggest that strength training alone prevents running injuries. Muscular weakness and poor mechanics are known to be present in injured runners. However, while strengthening programs improve symptoms, the poor mechanics are not necessarily altered without gait retraining.[14] In other words, strength training is most effective in combination with attention to gait and running form.

Q. What role does cross-training have in regards to running-related injuries? Can cross-training help avoid injuries?

A. Cross-training is an important factor in maintaining variability for the stresses applied to the lower extremities. While data does not exist regarding injury prevention, it is well accepted that varying your training program leads to increases in performance and reduction in repeated stress to the same anatomical structures.[15]

Q. How do I know if I have the following injuries and how do I treat them?

A. It is never best to self-diagnose or self-treat your running injuries. If you find that pain limits you from running for more than three consecutive running sessions or 1 week, you may need to seek the care of a sports medicine professional. A bout of rest is usually the best approach when injuries are minor or early in their course. Physicians and physical therapists specializing in sports, preferably running, can most efficiently guide you in your treatment and return to running. However, here are a few easy diagnostics and potential quick fixes.

Plantar fasciitis. Typical characteristics of plantar fasciitis are pain on the bottom of the heel bone close to the arch. The pain is usually most prevalent during the first few steps in the morning and may become less intense as you move around a bit. The best treatment for plantar fasciitis appears to be a 30-second extension stretch of the big toe before your foot hits the floor.

Achilles tendinitis. The Achilles tendon can hurt in two separate places: (1) in the middle just above the ankle bones and (2) where it connects to the heel bone. The tendon will hurt during running or walking and during standing. It may hurt more when you are barefoot or in low-profile shoes (sandals or flip-flops). Avoid stretching the tendon/calf until it is healed. Stretching too soon after apparent recovery will continue to damage the tissue. Massaging the calf muscle and a slight heel lift in the shoe will help the healing process.

"Shin splints." This is a term that encompasses a number of injuries that occur anywhere in the lower leg between the knee and ankle. Most often "shin splints" refers to medial tibial stress syndrome (MTSS). This condition is characterized by pain on the inside of the lower leg behind the shin bone. Most often, it will hurt after about 5 to 10 minutes of running and will increase in intensity. If severe, it will begin to hurt during walking. The best treatment for MTSS appears to be changing to supportive shoes, foot orthotics, and strengthening exercises targeting the muscles of the arch or lower leg.[16]

Stress fractures. Stress fractures can occur in the lower leg (tibia) and foot (metatarsals) and are usually related to overtraining. Stress fractures will present as focal points of pain, usually on the front of your shin bone (tibia) or on the top of your foot (metatarsal). The pain will likely increase over a period of a few weeks and become severe and sharp, especially during running or walking. Stress fractures require rest and usually a walking boot or crutches to take pressure off the limb. Once the stress fracture is resolved, a *gradual* return to running and gait analysis are necessary.

"Runner's knee." This is a term used to describe patellofemoral pain syndrome (PFPS). PFPS is characterized by pain just under the kneecap and can be present on the inside, outside, or both. The pain is present during running and when descending stairs or when rising from a chair after prolonged sitting. PFPS can be related to a number of factors. Hip weakness is common in individuals with PFPS. Therefore, strengthening of the hip abductors and rotators may be a good addition to your cross-training program.[17] (See the exercises in Chapter 12.) PFPS is also common in individuals with a low step count. Step counts under 160 steps have been shown to increase injury risk. Increasing your step count by 5 percent, if it is low, may be beneficial in reducing pain related to PFPS.[18]

Q. Do you recommend the Pose Method?

A. The Pose Method is a running technique developed by Nicholas Romanov, PhD, that focuses on soft landing and allowing gravity to help forward progression. It is characterized by a forward lean from the ankles, plus a slight bend in the knees and in the hips. There are a few studies demonstrating changes in biomechanics while using the Pose Method.[19] These characteristics are similar to those demonstrated during ChiRunning, midfoot running, and increases in stride frequency.

Personally, I do not recommend any specific form of running. Most runners have self-selected their running style based on their own personal energy demands and body characteristics. However, if a runner continues to get injured, changing mechanics may be an option. Recognize that there is no optimal running style for all runners, and no running style has been shown to reduce injury or improve performance.

Q. Please comment on barefoot running. Do you recommend it? Why or why not?

A. Barefoot running has received much attention in recent years, and we receive ample inquiry on its value. As noted above, no particular running style has been shown to reduce injury or improve performance, and barefoot running is no exception.

Advocates of barefoot running state that changing to a midfoot strike pattern during barefoot running reduces impacts. While this claim is accurate, many runners do not adopt a midfoot strike pattern when they run barefoot. In fact, studies have shown that 40 percent of runners still maintain a rear-foot strike pattern after training in barefoot conditions.[20]

Recent studies have also shown that barefoot running leads to large stresses in the foot bones contributing to stress reactions and fractures.[21] Advocates of barefoot running state there are increases in foot-muscle strength that occur. Even if barefoot running strengthens foot muscles—the evidence is sparse—there is no evidence to suggest that increasing muscle strength in the foot prevents injury or is even necessary.

Based on these findings, I see no strong justification for engaging in barefoot running. If a runner would like to run barefoot, my recommendation is to gradually adopt it over a 3- to 6-month period and use it sparingly. The best reason I can think of for barefoot running is that grass feels good on bare feet.

Q. What kind of running shoes do you recommend? Minimalist? Cushioned?

A. Running shoes can be a real conundrum. With so many shoe companies offering so many models that change every year, the decision can be mind-boggling.

No particular type of shoe has been shown to reduce injuries. Therefore, matching shoes to types of feet is not needed. In fact, large studies conducted with military recruits have demonstrated no decrease in running injuries when shoes were matched to foot type.[22] Additionally, recent data suggest the two most important factors in choosing shoes are fit and comfort.[23]

Simply buy the shoes that you like and make sure they feel good. Few individuals need extreme shoe types. For example, someone with a very rigid foot may benefit from a cushioned shoe *if* they are experiencing impact-related pain or injuries. Further, injured runners with very flexible feet may benefit from a stability or motion-control shoe in order to provide a stable platform for their feet or foot-orthotic devices. In my opinion, shoes receive too much credit and blame for successes and failures in running.

Q. Who should consider getting orthotics? Do you recommend the inserts that are often sold at running stores?

A. Orthotics are a brace that should be recommended by a sports medicine professional. Most people do not need foot orthoses. I recommend them for fewer than 20 percent of my running patients. The runners who typically benefit from foot orthoses have foot types that need a significant level of biomechanical control or cushioning.

Often, the devices that are sold in the running shoe stores are appropriate for most conditions. Custom devices are necessary only in cases where over-the-counter devices don't provide enough correction or do not fit the patient's foot. Like shoes, foot orthoses should fit and be comfortable. It is not acceptable to have expensive devices made for your feet and have them be so uncomfortable you can't wear them. You wouldn't buy $400 pants that were too tight or had one short leg. If you get custom devices, expect perfection.

Q. What surface is best for avoiding injury? Are running surfaces related to running-related injuries? Are some surfaces better for running than others?

A. This, for the most part, is an urban myth. There are no studies suggesting that surface plays any role in injury prevention. Based on laboratory-controlled studies, surface hardness does not result in increased or decreased impacts.[24] Unless you run on extremely soft surfaces, such as sand, there appears to be no difference in impacts between surfaces. So asphalt and concrete result in similar impacts. Then why do runners report that they feel better running on trails or on softer surfaces? The answer likely lies with the runner rather than the surface. Running on trails results in different running biomechanics, as more stability is required on uneven or softer surfaces. Impacts may be reduced with shorter, more purposeful steps and slower running speeds. Many runners report that running on trails provides relief from knee and hip irritation. The Furman University cross-country team and the professional runners that are part of Furman Elite train on a soft surface two or three times per week. However, as with shoes, comfort may be your best guide. If you feel better running on certain surfaces, do it!

Q. Any additional advice for how to avoid an injury?

A. Listen to your body. If you are feeling tired and sore, maybe an extra day off would be beneficial. If you are developing an increasingly

UP CLOSE AND PERSONAL

Robin began running in college to keep off the pizza pounds. She liked that running was a reliable, enjoyable, portable workout that she could do anywhere. Robin says that her running helped keep her sane during some major life events.

Name: Robin Politowicz
Age: 54
Occupation: Teacher
Hometown: Gainesville, FL
Race times: 5-K, 24:28 at age 53; half-marathon, 1:55:57
Age she began running: 19

For 20 years, she had an issue with stress fractures, as do many female runners. She realized she needed to vary her training and cut back from running 5 or 6 days per week. She began to strength train regularly and cross-train with swimming and biking.

Here is how Robin described her approach to running.

- I am a firm believer in the mental benefits of running and hard aerobic activity.
- I enjoy competition. It gives me motivation.
- I try to approach each race realistically and compete against myself instead of others.
- I admit that I find it is satisfying to place in my age group, and I am lucky that it happens pretty consistently.

Not many runners who have been running for 20 years achieve personal-best times in their fifties. For Robin, it was all about finding a way to train that would not leave her injured. Once she reduced her running frequency and added strength training to her workout regimen, she enjoyed injury-free running and faster race times. Robin, however, is not training less, but she is training more effectively. She is still getting plenty of aerobic exercise, which has enabled her to run personal-best times. Her changed behavior embodies the principles we are trying to promote.

painful knee or hip with every run, maybe it's time to reduce mileage or intensity. Watch your stress level. Increasing levels of stress increase injury propensity.

Q. What advice do you have for how to return to running after an injury? How do runners know when they can return to running?

A. Returning to running can be tricky. It is best to consult a therapist or medical professional who works with runners on a regular basis. Running requires a series of single-leg jumps from one leg to the other. The ability to control single-leg squats and landing is a good predictor of a successful return to running. At the VCU RUN LAB, we utilize a series of running-specific strength tests to determine readiness for return to running. Once runners master these tests, running begins progressively with a walk-run protocol that increases running time over 6 weeks and then increases running distance. Finally, running intensity is added as the final step to return to run. In short: Get strong, learn how to jump and land, walk-run, run farther, run faster.

CHAPTER 6

FINDING A TRAINING PROGRAM

WHEN I WALK ACROSS THE campus, I am often asked by colleagues and students which exercise is the best. I answer, "The one that you will do." To some extent, that's the same answer I offer as to which training program is best. It's the one that fits your lifestyle and personality. Maybe this chapter will help you determine that.

There is no shortage of running books and training programs. Many runners who have written to FIRST over the past 12 years have experimented with a variety of training programs. Sometimes the only way to know which program is best is through trial and error. In this chapter, I briefly describe the major features of the most popular training programs.

We are all unique subsets of one. We have unique physiologies and frames. We have different genes. Scientists can predict how runners as a class will respond to training quite well. However, how individuals respond to a training regimen will vary considerably.

Research studies show that some runners are high responders, meaning that their bodies adapt positively and rapidly to training.

On the other hand, other runners are low responders. They train hard for small improvements. There are even nonresponders, although they are rare.

You can be sure that you may respond more positively to one type of training as compared to another. We know from our coaching that we need to adjust training programs as we observe how runners respond to specific workouts.

Because of individual uniqueness, there is no universal best training program. All of us are left to figure out for ourselves which program is most effective. Unfortunately, there isn't any easy test for making that choice; you need to experiment. What is important is that you keep good training records so that you can assess how well you respond to different types of training. It is also important to pay attention to how much you enjoy the training.

Finding the right training program is a process. You can't assume that adopting the program of other runners who have had success will necessarily result in the optimal training method for you. On the other hand, if you have a training partner, you may want to consider a program that is mutually acceptable to both of you so you can continue the beneficial training relationship.

Using a training program for 12 to 16 weeks to prepare for one race may not be an adequate test of the program's effectiveness. Training is an ongoing process. Choose a program with the idea that it can be used for the long term. Give the training program a chance to determine if it is effective for you and your goals. It is important that you not only get the desired results from the program but that you also enjoy it.

Similarly, as you age you may find that you need a different training program. Typically, older runners need more recovery time and can tolerate less training volume.

Evolution and History of Distance-Running Training

A study of successful runners and coaches reveals that there is no one path to success for runners. Training methods over the past century have evolved, but along the way we see that there have been Olympic champions who utilized considerably different methods of training. Below are just a few examples.

Paavo Nurmi, the "Flying Finn," won gold medals at the 1924 Olympics in the 1500- and 5000-meter races. His training included lots of long walks of 6 miles in the morning with sprints from 80 to 800 meters in the afternoon. He carried a stopwatch on his run to become familiar with his pace and perceived exertion. He characterized his approach as what we describe today as "listening to your body." Nurmi, reflecting on his career, indicated that the greatest mistake he made in his training was too much long, slow running.[1]

Emil Zátopek is the only runner to win the 5000-meter, 10,000-meter, and Marathon in the same Olympics. The Czech accomplished that feat in the 1952 Games. Zátopek's basic training was interval training, alternating two basic interval workouts totaling 10 to 15 miles.[2] His interval workout of 10 x 200 meters and 50 x 400 meters has become a part of training folklore.

Franz Stampfl, an Austrian, is credited with introducing interval training as we know it today. Stampfl coached Roger Bannister, the first person to break 4 minutes for the mile. Stampfl trained Bannister to break the world record in the mile with a low-mileage, high-intensity regimen supported with days off for recovery.[3]

Contrasted with Stampfl's mechanistic and scientific approach was the eccentric Australian Percy Cerutty, who favored what he called Stotanism. Cerutty developed his holistic approach by combining stoic and Spartan principles. He preached going hard, withstanding pain, and showing no emotion. His outstanding pupil Herb Elliott won the 1500-meter at the 1960 Olympics. While Stampfl kept detailed and precise training records for Bannister, Cerutty would have Elliott running up sand dunes and along the beach. The two rival coaches utilized different approaches to training, but both produced world-record milers.[4]

Arthur Lydiard, the famed New Zealand coach, was responsible for introducing the idea of periodization and a strong endurance base. During the endurance-base phase, Lydiard insisted on 100-mile weeks for his runners. Lydiard coached Peter Snell, the great New Zealand runner, who won three Olympic gold medals in the 800-meter (1960 and 1964) and 1500-meter (1964) and broke the world record in the mile in 1962.[5]

Lydiard indirectly influenced the popularity of running in the United States through Bill Bowerman of Oregon. The revered Oregon coach visited Lydiard in New Zealand and was struck by how Lydiard had young and old citizens running using his "train, don't strain" philosophy. During the visit, Bowerman, 50 at the time, began jogging, a term he introduced to America. Bowerman was impressed with his personal results from easy running. When he returned to Eugene, he introduced folks young and old to jogging. He wrote a short pamphlet, *Jogging,* that contributed heavily to the popularity of running for the masses.[6]

Bowerman's hard-easy training principle brought a rational approach to training that shifted the emphasis away from excessive mileage to focused interval training. His impact on running also included his contributions to the development of running shoes, which led to the founding of Nike. Those who are old enough will remember the original "waffle trainers."

Jack Daniels, whom *Runner's World* magazine identified as "the world's greatest running coach," brought his training as an exercise physiologist to the study of running, most of it in the human performance laboratory. His studies examined the effects of various types of training on the development of fitness. Daniels focused on why a workout was included in one's training. He developed precise formulas for training based on science.[7] His approach focused on each of the major performance determinants—lactate threshold, aerobic capacity, and running economy—and how stress and recovery could contribute to improvement. As a college track and cross-country coach, Daniels led his teams to multiple national championships and produced more than a hundred All-Americans.

Features of Popular Training Programs

Runners have no shortage of popular training programs from which to choose for their race preparation. You can go online and read about the specific features associated with the various programs. Undoubtedly, there will always be new ones developed, but the primary features have many similar aspects. Most of these programs offer novice, intermediate, and advanced levels of training.

Some programs will have more appeal to a novice runner and others more attraction to a veteran runner. Some require more time and commitment than others. So how do you decide? Consider these questions when evaluating the features of a training program to help choose the best program for you.

How many miles per week are you currently running? What is the base training needed to start this program?

> ❭ A training program that begins with more miles than you are currently running may increase your risk of a running-related injury.

- A novice 5-K program may start with walking and introduce running with 1-minute walks.

- A veteran marathon training program commonly begins with 25 to 40 miles of weekly running.

- A base of 15 to 25 weekly miles is typically recommended to begin most marathon training programs.

What is the total weekly mileage of the program?

- This will vary from 15 to 25 miles per week for a 5-K program to 25 to 75 miles per week for marathon training programs.

When is your target event and how many weeks is the training program?

- Training programs can range from 12 to 30 weeks. Some of the length depends on whether you have already established base training.

- Modifying a training program to fit your race schedule may influence the effectiveness of the training program.

What is the distance of your longest run in the past 3 weeks?

- If the distance of the long run in the first week of the training program is farther than one of your most recent long runs, perhaps a few more weeks of base training would be wise.

- You want the training program to improve your current running fitness, not wear you out.

What is the longest run included in the training program?

- A 5-K program may include a long run of 3 to 6 miles.

- Marathon programs generally include long runs of 15 to 20 miles.

- How many of these long marathon training runs are included in the program?

- Some will build to one 20-mile run. Others may include a weekly long run of 20 miles every other week.

- A few marathon programs have long runs that exceed 20 miles.

Does the training program include speed training?

- What type?
  - Track repeats? Specific distances and paces usually run on a measured track or path.
  - Fartlek? A recommendation of interspersing some fast running into one of your regular runs.
  - Tempo runs? Running at a prescribed pace or perceived level of exertion for 15 to 30 minutes.

How many speed workouts are there per week?

- Some programs include no speed workouts, and others might have two per week.

How many days per week do you have available to exercise?

- For a training program to be effective, you want the program to use your available training time optimally.

- If you are able to exercise 4 days per week, then a 5-day-per-week training program may be frustrating.

How many days per week of running?

❭ Training programs vary from 3 to 7 days per week of running.

Does the program Include cross-training?

❭ What type?

- Cycling, biking, rowing, elliptical trainers, stairclimbers, others?
- Do you have access to the types of exercise included in the training program?

❭ How often?

- Recommendations vary from 0 to 2 days per week.

Does the program provide intensity recommendations for each workout?

❭ Are the recommendations general—hard, moderate, easy?

- Some programs designate the intensity of the workout by your perceived exertion.

❭ Are there specific time targets for each workout?

- Some programs indicate a target time or pace for the workout.
- Are your target times realistic? Attempting to complete workouts at paces faster than your current fitness supports will increase your risk of a running-related injury.

❭ How are the target times determined?

- Some programs use your fitness level as determined by a specific workout time, a recent race time, or a goal race time for selecting your target workout times.

- Some programs base target times on goal finish times. There are pitfalls to this approach.

Does the training program include nonrunning workouts?

❭ Are there recommendations for resistance training?
- Some programs are just running workouts. Others emphasize strength training as part of the training program.

❭ Are there recommendations for stretching?
- Some programs include specific stretches with guidelines for their inclusion in the training program.

These questions will guide you in evaluating whether a program fits your current fitness level and goals. They will also help you assess whether the time and energy demands of the program are compatible with your responsibilities and interests.

Are the FIRST Training Programs the Best?

As the cofounder of the FIRST training programs, I am asked why the FIRST training programs are better than others. I have never said that the FIRST training programs are better than other training programs. We developed the FIRST training programs to assist runners of all ages and abilities to achieve their goals. In particular, we did so to promote running as a healthy, lifelong physical activity.

We have assisted thousands of runners since the founding of FIRST in 2003. Many have used the program to achieve personal best times, including qualifying for the Boston Marathon. More important, many runners have been able to run injury-free using the program after being unable to do so with other training programs.

FIRST is often criticized for being a minimalist program, and in fact, our program embraces the philosophy of stressing quality over quantity. Why? Many runners do not have physiques that will tolerate the frequency and duration of running practiced by elite runners. That is why the FIRST program substitutes cross-training for additional run days.

UP CLOSE AND PERSONAL

I was invited to India to deliver a series of talks on running and training. While I was there, Shiv served as my daily guide. He arranged my appearances with clubs and media and met me at the hotel with the driver and car. He was eager to learn all he could about training. He had been running for 3 years, but his training knowledge was limited.

Name: Shiv Shankar Kosgi

Age: 31

Occupation: Operations manager, Hyderabad Runners Society

Hometown: Hyderabad, India

Race times: Marathon, 3:50

Age he began running: 25

I invited Shiv to come to the United States to spend 2 weeks with us at FIRST. He describes his visit to the FIRST Lab and Furman University as a once-in-a-lifetime experience. He became a subject for all the lab assessments. He was also able to sit in on lectures, observe coaching and laboratory testing, participate in training sessions, and even run a marathon.

Here is how Shiv reported that his FIRST experience improved his running.

- It helped me understand the scientific methods and techniques of training.
- FIRST sessions helped me understand the importance of becoming stronger for injury prevention.
- I learned about different types of training to include in my marathon training (e.g., intervals, tempo, hills, long run).

The distinctive features of the FIRST training programs available in *Runner's World Run Less, Run Faster* include 3 days of running and 2 days of aerobic cross-training. While the running component of the FIRST training program may be fewer days than many training programs, the total amount of exercise is similar to other training programs.

In the FIRST marathon training program, the long runs are run closer to marathon pace than the paces recommended by other training programs. I believe that running the long runs closer to

- Drills had never been a part of my training. I added them to improve my running posture. I have improved a lot in terms of cadence and running form.
- I now know the importance of rest and nutrition.

Shiv returned to India, followed the FIRST training program, and, for the first time, broke 4 hours in the marathon. He reported that he not only finished with a PR of 3:50:01, but that it was also not so difficult for him to achieve this target because of his proper, disciplined training.

Shiv recently resigned from his IT job to become the operations manager of the Hyderabad Runners Society. It's a running club that in only 6 years has reached a membership of more than 3,000 runners. Its growth has paralleled the growing interest in running and fitness among the expanding middle class in India.

Shiv provides members of the Hyderabad Runners Society with structured workouts. He posts workouts on social media for members of the club. They train at sites all over the city of 6 million, using the workout of the day. He includes run workouts, strength-training exercises, and stretches for the runners. This structured approach has resulted in vast running performance improvements for club members.

Hyderabad runners have become more disciplined in terms of following a training plan. The number of people taking up running for fitness in Hyderabad is growing every year. Shiv's own running benefited from his expanded knowledge and experiences, and all of Hyderabad is benefiting from his commitment to the health and wellness of its citizens.

marathon pace prepares the runner for the demands on race day (the principle of specificity).

Since many of the runners who follow our program are busy professionals, they often do not have the time and energy to run more often than 3 days per week. I have been running 3 days per week for 25 years. I like the variety of doing different activities; so does my body.

We hear regularly from runners who tell us that they enjoy the "3plus2"—three weekly runs and two cross-training workouts—training program because it fits their busy lives. Aging runners tell us the programs work well for them because they need more recovery days between runs.

CHAPTER **7**

DO I NEED A COACH OR TRAINING PARTNER?

WHEN I BEGAN DISTANCE RUNNING and road racing in the mid-1970s, it was rare to see a group running together—or even a pair of runners. In the small towns of southern West Virginia and southwestern Virginia, I rarely saw another runner. Highways were the only options for distance running, and the coal trucks did not appreciate my efforts to improve my cardiorespiratory endurance. They definitely did not like sharing the road.

In the late '70s, my brother and I moved to nearby towns, which permitted us to meet and train together, and I discovered the synergistic effect of running with a partner. I became intrigued with the discovery that running beside someone seemed to create or transfer energy from one to another.

As I have mentioned, for the past 35 years I have been fortunate to share nearly all my training runs with my coauthor Scott and/or my brother, Don. We are not just training partners—we are also one another's informal coaches. It helps to have someone who observes your training and racing offer advice. Often someone else can better assess whether you are doing too much, too little, or too much of the same.

Many runners have discovered the value of running with others, while some still welcome "the loneliness of the long-distance runner." You are more likely to see pairs or groups today than the lone runner. Most runners probably run with others on a local bike path, with a group doing a track workout, or on a treadmill in a busy fitness center. Running clubs, shoe stores, fitness clubs, and YMCAs regularly sponsor running groups that meet at regular times for training runs.

Run Alone or with a Partner?
Consider Some of the Benefits of Running with Others

Accountability. Running with others holds you accountable on a cold, wet morning when you would rather stay in bed. When others are expecting you, you are more likely to show up. Having a training partner or being part of an exercise group is the variable that will most likely lead to sticking with an exercise program.

Consistency. The primary key to improvement is consistency. Having a regular training schedule and training with others toward a common goal contributes to consistency.

Motivation. Running with others motivates you. When you see others push themselves, you are more likely to make that extra effort. Many times I have commented after a workout that I would not have done the last two repeats had others quit, but if they were going to do them, I was, too.

Variety. Running with others provides variety. Running with others encourages you to try new workouts, distances, and races. Running alone can limit your experiences and prevent you from improving as a runner. A mixture of workouts can help make you a more balanced runner.

Group pressure. Running with others creates an excitement that helps you run faster than you thought you could on your own. According to social psychologists, there are psychological benefits that come from running with a group. Social facilitation is the tendency for people to do better when in the presence of others. In other words, there is an improvement in performance when the eyes of the group are on you. So when running with others, you may not realize how fast you are actually running; you keep up when you might have otherwise slowed down if running alone.

Camaraderie. Enduring friendships are made during the many miles shared. Training for a race is hard; embarking on a challenge with others makes it seem a little less daunting. Running with a partner gives you the chance to complain about your job, the weather, even your spouse. Everyone needs a listening friend.

Safety. Personal safety is a bigger issue these days. Just like the adage "never swim alone," you are safer when you run with others.

Consider Some of the Benefits of Running Alone

"Me" time. Life is crazy busy. Among chirping cell phones, pinging e-mails, talkative coworkers, and a crazy family schedule, it is often tough to find a second for "me" time. After a long day at work, there is nothing quite as cathartic as a long run outside by yourself. The stress of life seems to dissolve soon after you hit the pavement.

No pressure. No specific distance, no specific pace, no specific course. On a solo run you can simply listen to how your body feels. Running without regard to where, when, or how fast can be very liberating. The sense of freedom when going out for a run by yourself can be tough to match.

Your pace. Unless you have a training partner with a similar fitness level, you will either be forced to run too hard or too easily. To counteract that, some days you may wish to run alone so you can run at just the right pace for you.

Postinjury return to running. When you run on your own, it is easier to pay attention to your form and effort. Running by yourself can be especially important if you are returning to running after an injury and need to listen to your body to avoid a setback. Listening to your body is important and sometimes easier to do when you run alone.

Competition-free. As runners, most of us have a competitive side, but training runs need not always be a race. However, some partners always make a training run a race. Everyone knows that runner who has to be positioned one step ahead. Yes, it is annoying.

Flexibility. Having a plan is a good idea; however, having the freedom to modify when and where you run can be done more easily when you are running alone.

Meditation. Running alone can be meditative. You can think and concentrate or completely clear your mind and let it spin freely. Running alone also helps you achieve "flow," defined by psychologist Mihaly Csikszentmihalyi in *Flow: The Psychology of Optimal Experience* as the state of complete absorption to the point where everything else simply falls away.[1] Achieving flow is almost always a solo endeavor.

Race-day preparation. Ultimately, running is an individual activity. Getting to the finish line on race day is something only you can do. Solo runs prepare you to be self-sufficient on race day: You'll get accustomed to knowing your body (when to hydrate and fuel) and, more important, finding and maintaining your pace without relying on your training partner's help.

Alone and Together

With so many advantages to both running on your own and running with others, it is smart to do some of each. An individual runner might want to pair with friends for speedwork and join others for company on long runs. Group runners can split off from their buddies in order to maintain their tempo pace for a quality workout. Consider these suggestions for the different kinds of runs.

Track workouts seem so much easier when you do them with others. We often comment, "I wouldn't have run those times if I had been out here by myself." Join your partner or running group for the warmup and drills, but once your track workout starts, run your paces and avoid making the workout a race. Once you have finished your track workout, join the others for a cooldown and discussion of the workout. However, when you are training with someone of comparable ability and similar goals, each can help push the other to achieve the mutual target time.

Tempo runs can be tough, but knowing your running partner is doing the same run can keep you motivated. Join your partner or running buddies for the warmup, but run your tempo pace for the designated distance. We stagger the start of our tempo runs so that we all tend to catch up with one another with half a mile to go. Knowing running buddies are ahead of you or behind you helps you maintain your pace during the last part of a tempo run. The cooldown is a good time to compare actual paces to target paces.

Running with others certainly seems to make the miles of a long run go by more quickly, even when ability and fitness levels are different. Easing into a long run, you can run with your partners for the first couple of miles. As each of you finds his or her target pace for the run, you may separate, but knowing that others are on the same course still makes it easier. You may even regroup at intersections or at your designated rehydration location. You can join together for the cooldown and postrun refueling.

Do I Need a Coach?

Andrew Metzger, a 47-year-old neurosurgeon from Albuquerque, New Mexico, had not achieved his goal of a sub-3-hour marathon, and he felt that time was closing in on him. Fifty was just around the corner, and he knew that his times would plateau and eventually begin to slow. His battles over the past 5 years had been more with injuries than aging. Or maybe aging was contributing to the injuries. Regardless of the culprit preventing him from completing a marathon training cycle without an injury, he needed to find a solution before the inevitable consequences of aging kept him from ever becoming a 2-something marathoner.

Andrew had read numerous books about training and had an idea about which training program would work best for him. However, as a physician with a busy work schedule, he thought that finding a coach who could tailor his training specifically to his running history and his physiological parameters would increase the likelihood of achieving his goal of a sub-3-hour marathon.

These days it is common for a coach and runner to develop a long-distance relationship through electronic communication and never actually meet in person. However, Andrew thought that meeting his coach would enable the coach to be more familiar with him and better able to create an individualized plan for success. Andrew traveled to Furman University to have a lab assessment and to meet Scott Murr. With that meeting, they began a 3-year coach-runner relationship.

Scott guided Andrew through five sub-3-hour marathons, with a personal best of 2:52 at Boston. Andrew admits that it is likely that he could self-coach reasonably well after learning from Scott, but he continues to work with Scott. Here is his explanation for why he continues having a coach.

> The accountability of having to report on my progress each week helps keeps me motivated, even when a busy work schedule or bad weather work against this. My window to exercise on weekdays is before work, so I am often training at 5:30 a.m. in the dark and cold.

> Target paces are important in training, and it can be difficult for me to objectively choose the optimal level of intensity for different workouts. I think having an experienced coach oversee training and progress is a much better way to optimize training.

> Invariably, I have disruptions to my training schedule due to long work hours, travel, illness, and injury. Scott is able to modify my training to work effectively around these disruptions and still guide me to marathon PRs.

> Scott has been able to develop for me an effective race strategy. He has assisted me not only with the physical aspects of racing but also with how to mentally approach different phases of the marathon, and this has proven quite helpful.

Andrew's success demonstrates the value of a coach. His analysis explains how having a coach has contributed to his success.

Andrew gained confidence in Scott's advice because he had initial success under Scott's guidance. Having confidence in your training is valuable. It enabled Andrew to perform each workout without wondering if he was doing what was best. It removed the doubt about whether he was doing too much or too little.

The confidence that Andrew had in his coach also encouraged him to embrace Scott's racing strategy. There is nothing worse in a marathon than wondering if your pace is too fast or too slow. Andrew followed his planned race strategy, which most likely led him to run more relaxed without the mental stress associated with questioning whether he was running a smart race.

UP CLOSE AND PERSONAL

In high school and college, John was a standout track athlete. He finished second in the NCAA Division III 5000-meter track national championships. Soon after graduating from college, John ran a 2:37 marathon. He did not continue training and running with the same regularity while completing his graduate studies and during his journalism career as a TV news producer. From age 25 to age 50, he ran sporadically and without a systematic training program.

Name: John Armstrong
Age: 62
Occupation: Professor of communications
Hometown: Greenville, SC
Race times: Marathon, 3:24 at age 60; 2:37 (PR) at age 22
Age he began running: 15

After back surgery in 2011, John was able to resume consistent training in 2014. He realized that he could not avoid injury and irritation to his back if he ran daily. He conferred with Scott and me and decided to try following the FIRST marathon training program.

Here is how John described his experience with running 3 days per week.

- In 2014–2015, I used the FIRST running program to improve my marathon time from 3:47 to 3:24 over a span of just 5 months.

Consider the Benefits of Having a Coach

The difference between a dream and a goal is a plan. Accomplishing a goal typically requires two main components: a structured program and consistent training. In general, every runner benefits from a combination of miles and consistency in training. Most runners have a hard time taking their emotions out of their training. Consequently, runners often fall into the trap of thinking that "more is better." A coach can provide a more balanced perspective

- The two marathons were run on courses of very similar difficulty and in almost identical weather conditions.
- I not only qualified for the Boston Marathon with my 3:24 but also achieved another goal by qualifying for the New York City Marathon.
- My training program centered on FIRST's 3-day-per-week workouts.
- I also dropped my weight by following FIRST's dietary recommendations, and I did only light exercise on the days in between workouts—usually 1- to 2-mile walks.
- I was able to sustain the FIRST training program without any serious physical ailments. I attribute this to the emphasis on recovery in the FIRST program.

Even at age 60, John still had a robust cardiorespiratory system and an efficient stride. He needed a plan that would enable him to avoid his repetitive orthopedic injuries. John also wanted a training plan that fit with his busy schedule but would enable him to race competitively in his age group. The 3 days of running along with regular stretching and strength exercises gave him a fresh and renewed approach to running.

and prevent a runner from falling into the trap of extremes. And the trap of extremes usually leads to injury.

If you want to start running or keep running and remain healthy and fit for as long as you can, getting a running coach can be more valuable than buying the right pair of running shoes. Because running is an individual sport, runners tend to think that they do not need a coach. A running coach is just as important for middle-of-the-pack runners as for those racing for the win.

When it comes to running, objectivity matters. When left up to their own analysis, most runners will push too hard (increasing their risk of injury and failing to elicit the appropriate training response) or not run hard enough (failing to elicit the training stimulus needed to improve). A coach provides objectivity.

A good coach will see the whole picture and consider the multiple demands of your life, family, work, illness, and training. Your coach can develop an efficient plan that benefits you the most without wasted time or energy in workouts you may not need. Coaches offer feedback and can make adjustments to training as needed. A coach takes guesswork out of your training. A coach can reduce the risk of injury with a plan that includes proper rest and recovery—something self-coached runners often neglect.

Coaches encourage you to determine if your aspirations are realistic. They identify what it will take to meet your objectives and can outline the path toward accomplishing them. The more defined and measurable goals are, the easier they are to achieve. A coach provides accountability and keeps you on target.

Coaches keep you consistent. Distance running is a long-term sport, so runners need to remind themselves that results do not happen overnight or even in weeks or a few months. One study suggested that one-on-one personal training is effective not only for changing attitudes toward physical activity but also for increasing the amount of time participants spend being physically active.[2] Consistency is the key.

Coordinating your runs with a partner or a group certainly helps you stay on track for a challenging goal or race. Most runners start running because of a specific objective: to lose weight or to accept a challenge with a friend or coworker (finish a 5-K, a half-marathon, or even a marathon). Whether they will admit it or not, most runners have goals. While numerous training programs are available in magazines, books, and online that can be effective for reaching your objective, a customized training program may offer additional benefits, and a running coach or a trusty training partner can be an added ingredient in the recipe for accomplishing your goal.

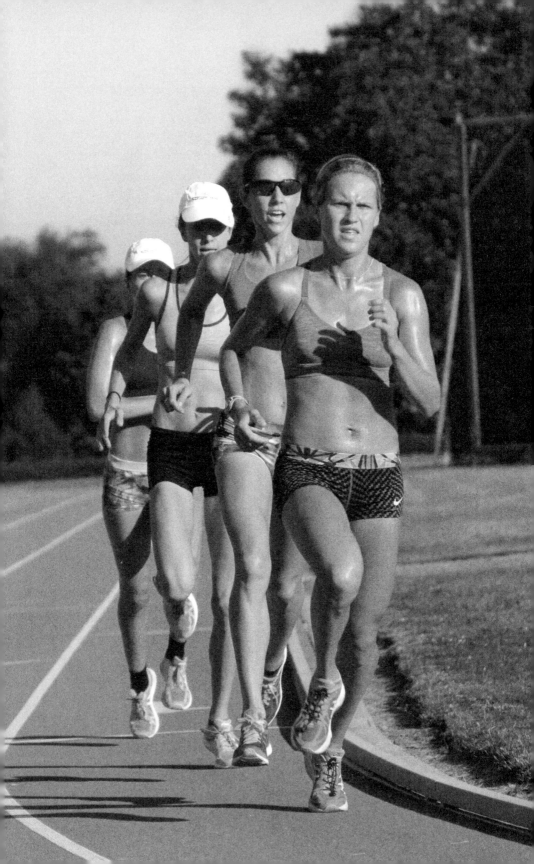

CHAPTER 8

SMART PACING IS ESSENTIAL FOR SMART TRAINING AND RACING

ONE OF THE QUESTIONS MOST frequently asked of us is, "What should my goal race time be?" It is also the most difficult question to answer. Even when the request is accompanied by detailed training and racing data, which most often it is not, providing the runner with a realistic and optimal target finish time is difficult. Multiple variables influence race performance.

Many runners select goal times that are unrealistic given their training but are appealing because those times are nice round numbers. It is fine to want to break 4 hours or qualify for Boston, but only if you have trained consistently at the appropriate pace. Most running coaches and exercise physiologists recommend that you run your race at a constant pace, even though runners are tempted to start out fast to put some "time in the bank." This pacing strategy generally backfires and leads to a less-than-optimal performance.

Even pacing is challenging and not often achieved by runners. In particular, few marathoners run their race at a constant pace. Small deviations in pace in shorter races—5-Ks and 10-Ks—may not yield the optimal performance, but their impact on the finish time is minimal for a well-trained runner. However, for the marathoner, deviations from even pacing usually have a large, negative impact on finish time.

How, then, should a runner decide what pace is realistic and optimal? It is always disappointing to have to tell a runner that based on her past performances, a sub-4-hour finish is unrealistic. She tells us she has been trying to hit it for years and has gotten close. Her last marathon was 4:06. Six minutes! Shouldn't she be able to shave those off? However, 6 minutes translates to 14 seconds per mile. As most of us know, running 14 seconds per mile faster for 26 miles is a stiff challenge. Doing so would require a significant improvement in fitness. If she is a veteran runner who is quite possibly running close to her potential, that size of improvement would require significant changes in training, perhaps with nutrition, body-weight, and pacing strategy.

Runners want to know their absolute fastest possible time. That is a thorny question with intricate factors making a simple answer impossible.

The Importance of Training at an Effective Effort Level

Those familiar with the FIRST training programs in *Runner's World Run Less, Run Faster* use our tables to know exactly what pace to use on each of their runs based on their current fitness level. Our training principle is that you must gradually increase stress; this causes the body to adapt to an overload. The training principle of progressive overload requires that you run a little faster or a little farther to stimulate your body to adapt to the increased workload. That stress is followed by a recovery period that allows your body to adjust to the increased stress. Then, continuing the process, you add a little more speed and/or a little more distance. This gradual progression of increased stress is the effective and safe way to improve fitness.

To get faster, you need to run faster. It seems obvious. But each run must serve a purpose. Each run needs to be performed at an intensity that provides just enough stress on the body to make it adapt without suffering injury or being unable to perform subsequent training workouts.

When we initially question runners about their training, we often hear that they do all of their runs at approximately the same pace or effort level and often for the same distance. Often they are even running the same routes. We tell them they need to shake it up. You need shorter, faster, more-intense runs to increase speed and longer runs to build endurance.

Finding the right training pace, one that is consistent with your fitness level, becomes even more important for the aging runner. Whereas younger runners can push the limits on their paces and do it frequently, older runners are more prone to injury and need more time to recover from hard training sessions.

The Importance of Racing at an Effective Pace

The textbook recommendation for optimal pacing based on energy conservation is even pacing. Exercise physiology researcher Stephen Seiler, PhD, dean of the Faculty of Health and Sport Sciences at University of Agder, Kristiansand, Norway, explains that poor pacing accelerates lactic acid accumulation, dehydration, and glycogen depletion, which will prevent marathoners from achieving their goal finish times.[1] He adds that maintaining a constant speed is necessary to achieve peak performance.

Some coaches propose that just because even pacing seems to be the optimal pacing strategy for the world's best runners does not mean it is necessarily the best pacing strategy for non-elite runners. Some recognize that the more modest a runner's fitness level is, the more likely it is that he will achieve his fastest time by running somewhat aggressively in the first half of a race and then "hanging on" in the second half.

This strategy is appealing to new marathoners, since if you have trained well and tapered, when you get to the starting line you are amped up and will find it easy to go out fast and believe you can hold it. Only after crashing and burning in a number of races will you realize that the first half should feel easy. We believe that going out too fast is a recipe for failure.

Some advocate running a "negative split." Tim Noakes, MD, who does not believe in the "time cushion" approach, argues that you should always aim to run the second half of a race, regardless of distance, slightly faster than the first.[2] The problem is that a negative split is really hard to do, unless you just sandbag the first half, which will not enable you to run your optimal time.

Bob Glover and Pete Schuder caution in *The New Competitive Runner's Handbook* that if your half-marathon split is more than 2 minutes faster than half of your target marathon time, then you have blown your marathon optimal time and will suffer for it over the last few miles.[3] Marathoners commonly refer to a dramatic slowing of pace in the marathon as "hitting the wall." David Costill, PhD, states that "hitting the wall" is simply a matter of poor pacing.

Dr. Seiler reports that for each second gained by running faster than optimal pace in the first half of a race, 2 seconds are lost in the second half due to premature fatigue.[4]

At FIRST, even though we recognize that in theory an even pace is recommended, we suggest that marathoners build a "little time" cushion for those last few miles. This little time cushion requires running a marathon pace that is slightly faster than planned for some of the miles. Note that we say "slightly." Our definition of marathon even pacing is that your two half-marathon splits do not differ by more than 2 minutes.

Here is how we suggest pacing a marathon to the runners we coach. Run the first couple of miles at planned marathon pace (PMP) or even 5 seconds slower per mile than PMP. Lock into PMP for the next 8 miles. At 10 miles, run 5 to 10 seconds per mile faster than PMP for the next 10 miles. That provides you with 50 to 100 seconds as a cushion for the last 6 miles, which can mean running 8 to 16 seconds per mile slower as you begin to tire. That provides some mental relief as you get to 20 miles and know that you have a little leeway as the running gets much tougher mentally as well as physically.

How to Select a Realistic Pace

Marathoners who fail to achieve their goal finish time almost immediately begin to question their preparation and training. In many cases, their preparation was good and appropriate, but they may have been unlucky because one of the many variables that come into play with an endurance event was not ideal that day. Frequently, it is temperature or humidity that prevents a runner from reaching a realistic target goal. However, setting an unrealistic marathon goal finish time—even one that is just a couple minutes too fast—will lead to a too-fast early pace that will undermine good preparation and great effort.

Selecting a realistic finish time should include a thorough review of your training and race results. Recent race times at different distances are valuable predictors of marathon times. There are many tables and online calculators that enable you to enter a 5-K, 10-K, or half-marathon time and predict a marathon finish time. As you might expect, a half-marathon time will be a better predictor for the marathon than a 5-K time.

The difficulty of the race course and the race-day weather forecast must also be considered in your determination of a realistic race pace. Hilly courses, temperatures over 60 degrees, and high humidity will not lead to optimal race performances.

Also valuable in choosing the right marathon pace are your long training run paces. You should develop a sense of what pace is realistic, assuming that you have been doing long runs of 10 to 20 miles for 12 to 16 weeks. We recommend that you run your long efforts with at least a few miles at the finish or, even better, the entire run at goal marathon pace.

By running at marathon pace during a long run of 2 to 3 hours, you can at least determine if it is feasible to consider running the full marathon at that pace.

While Don, Scott, and I often finish our long runs at marathon pace, I have to confess that after a long training run, I have difficulty imagining another 6 to 10 miles at an even faster pace. It is not easy to comprehend the benefits of a taper. The same pace that was difficult on those long training runs typically feels much easier on race day due to the taper and the exhilaration associated with the long-awaited event.

How Likely Is It That Runners Will Achieve an Even Pace?

How many runners actually maintain an even pace? In 2001, my brother, Don, and I analyzed nearly 50,000 marathon finish times from the Chicago Marathon and the New York City Marathon to answer the question. The Chicago Marathon course is flat, and the New York City Marathon is relatively flat with a few rolling hills. Neither marathon had extreme weather conditions in 2000. Both of the races had a large number of runners, computer-chip timing that provided net half-marathon splits, and a broad national and international representation. For those reasons, we decided that they would be good marathons to see how many runners achieved an even pace.

What we found was that approximately 5 percent of the marathoners in the two marathons had half-marathon split times that did not deviate more than 1 minute. Furthermore, slightly more than 10 percent had half-marathon split times that did not deviate more than 2 minutes. We consider these even-pace marathons. Consequently, nearly 90 percent of the finishers in the country's two largest marathons did not achieve their potential.[5]

It is unknown how many of the marathoners attempted to run even splits. Even many veteran marathoners are not confident enough of their ability to sustain a constant pace for the entire distance, particularly over the last 6 miles, to employ an even-pace strategy. Marathoners tend to cling to the notion that time gained in the first half can offset the time lost over the last 6 miles.

You are likely to have read about elite marathoners running even or negative splits. Remember, elite marathoners are running for slightly over 2 hours. Many of us can maintain even pacing for 2 hours. Elite marathoners train 120 or more miles per week as compared to less than half or a third of that distance for most of us non-elite runners. Running 26 miles is a fraction of their weekly mileage as opposed to being closer to non-elites' total weekly mileage. That is why running even splits is not unusual for elite marathoners.

Will Using a Pacing Group Help Achieve My Goal Time?

In 1995, at some of the major marathons, *Runner's World* magazine began providing pacers to help runners qualify for the 100th Boston Marathon in 1996.[6] The pacing program was received so well that many marathons now offer pacing groups. Generally, runners do not need to sign up or pay. They simply fall in behind pacers who carry signs with the target marathon finish time (e.g., 3:00, 3:10, 3:30, 4:00, etc.) and run at the constant minutes-per-mile pace necessary to produce the target finish time.

The 2001 Chicago Marathon organizers supplied us with pacing group data so that we could analyze the success of the pacing group participants. Overall, 24.9 percent of the pacing group participants finished within 5 minutes of their goals.[7]

Why did more than 75 percent of the pacing group participants fail to finish within 5 minutes of their goal time? Given that a pacer running at a constant pace led the pacing group participants, can it be surmised that the low rate of success for pacing group participants was due to the selection of overly ambitious goal times?

We felt it would be interesting to know if those who joined a pacing group expected to run the entire distance with the pacer or if they planned to use the pacer to reach an intermediate mile marker at a target time. In the latter case, the marathoner's strategy may have included running a different pace over the last part of the race.

To answer our own question about the intentions of pacing group participants, we surveyed the 2001 Chicago Marathon pacing group participants. It is interesting that 36.5 percent of the males and 36.6 percent of the females indicated that they did not intend to stay with the pacer the entire distance. The rationale for forming pacing groups is to help runners maintain a constant pace throughout the marathon. Despite the advice of most trainers, marathoners commonly develop and employ non-even pacing strategies. Over a third of the runners reported that they intended to run a different pace than the pacing group they joined. Apparently, over a third of those joining pacing groups are using the pacer to help achieve a target time for only a segment of the marathon. Interestingly, more than 84 percent of the respondents said they planned to join a pacing group in their next marathon.

Pacing groups continue to be popular, and their availability at half-marathons and marathons is widespread. The Minnesota Pacers, an experienced race team of more than 20 runners, has been providing pacing services for races since 2010. Each of the team members leads pacing groups for 10 to 15 races per year. When I asked Sam Ryder, the owner of the team, how many runners stick with the pacer for the entire race, he said that only about 10 percent of the runners who join a pacing group will run every mile stride for stride with the pacer. He responded further that typically 20 percent of the runners will not last past mile 10. He commented that those runners had set an unrealistic goal. Another 40 percent will fall off the pace before mile 20, he said, describing that group as not properly trained or just having a bad day. Of the 40 percent of runners who are with the pacer at 20 miles, some will run ahead of the pacer and finish a minute or more ahead of the pacer, and some will not be able to stay with the pacer.

In the marathons I've run over the last 3 years, most of the pacing groups have dwindled to just a few runners by the end. One factor that contributes to pacing group disintegration is that runners are forced to choose a group that is either slightly too fast or too slow. Runners often ask me which pacing group they should follow when their goal finish time falls between two pacing groups. For example, consider that we have determined that 3:35 to 3:40 is the runner's target time, and the race offers 3:30 and 3:45 pacing groups. In that case, the marathoner should not join either pacing group. One group would have the runner too fast, and that would lead to disaster later in the race. The other group would have the runner too slow, with too much time to make up once leaving the pacing group.

Nonetheless, we recognize that having someone set the pace is helpful. As long as you can find a pacing group that matches your target time, we endorse having the pacer and the group assist you to the finish line.

Pacing Recommendation Question

A question I often receive from runners has to do with multiple goals for their next marathon. The common scenario includes runners who want to qualify for Boston but also wish to run under a specific time or a personal best that is faster than the Boston qualifying time. The question: What pace should I run? My answer: Which goal is more important? Are you willing to risk not qualifying for Boston by going for the specific time that is better than the Boston qualifying standard?

The answer to the query is a highly individualized decision. If the runner is confident that a Boston qualification can be achieved at another time, or if maybe a Boston qualification has been achieved in the past, the runner may be willing to take the risk of

UP CLOSE AND PERSONAL

Angela conducts an outdoor fitness business that has a heavy focus on running. Each year she trains more than 150 runners for the Gold Coast Marathon. On a weekly basis, Angela coordinates programs for a large client base of more than 4,500 people.

Angela has been recognized as the Australian Institute of Personal Trainers Educator of the Year, and her business, Savvy Fitness, was named by the Australian Health and Fitness Industry as the Personal Training Business of the Year.

Name: Angela Saville
Age: 37
Occupation: Fitness professional
Hometown: Wollongong, NSW, Australia
Race times: 5-K, 18:55; 10-K, 38:40; half-marathon, 1:26; marathon, 3:13
Age she began running: 23

Scott and I enjoyed working with Angela when she came to visit us at Furman. Here is how Angela described her running using our training concepts.

- I was running 5 or 6 times per week and not paying much attention to my training paces when I came across the *Run Less, Run Faster* training program in 2012 while doing research on run programming.
- I particularly loved the concept of quality over quantity.
- I decided to see if I could successfully achieve my goal time while reducing my running to three sessions per week.
- I followed the plan strictly.
- There was an excitement of not really knowing what I was capable of but finally having something to guide me.
- The marathon performance itself was a success!
- My goal was a sub-3:15:00 and I ran a 3:13.

Once Angela began training at a pace that stimulated a fitness adaptation, her running times improved greatly. In this chapter, we emphasized the importance of training at the appropriate intensity.

After Angela experienced personal success, she introduced training programs with specific target pacing to the runners she coaches. She recently reported that all the runners she trained for the Sydney Marathon improved their time from their previous marathon, and half of them had personal-best times.

not qualifying for Boston by going for the more ambitious time goal. In particular, if the runner feels that he is in the best shape of his life and this might be the best opportunity ever to run that personal time goal, the runner might be willing to take the risk of falling apart from choosing a pace that is too ambitious. If, on the other hand, the runner has never qualified for Boston and that is the overarching goal, then a more conservative pace would be recommended to ensure that goal.

Selection of training and racing paces requires a scientific approach. However, be aware that even the most scientific analysis might not have the refinement and specificity to produce the optimal performance. Most runners find that a certain amount of trial and error is needed to determine their optimal pace. Part of the intrigue of racing the marathon distance is the uncertainty associated with the results.

CHAPTER 9

EAT SMART FOR THE LONG RUN

REMEMBER THE DAYS WHEN WE ran in cotton shirts? Remember those short, silky Dolphin shorts? Adidas SL 72s and Etonic Street Fighters that turned your socks blue? Race bibs without chips? Remember when we did not carry water? Remember when there were no energy bars? Or gels? Or sports drinks at aid stations? Or when aid stations were at 5-mile intervals in marathons?

When runners come to the FIRST retreats and get the results of their body composition scans, we often must have an uncomfortable conversation about how their weight prevents them from getting faster. I explain that the science of nutrition is complex, but the adoption of a healthy eating plan is simple.

Over the last 40 years, sports and exercise scientists have conducted numerous nutritional studies in an effort to determine how to best enhance human performance through food and drink consumption. Hundreds of books have been written about which dietary plan is healthiest. The study of nutrition and sports nutrition continues to grow.

In 1975, the American College of Sports Medicine (ACSM), in a position statement on the prevention of heat injuries, recommended that the rule prohibiting the administration of fluids during the first 10 kilometers of a marathon race should be amended to permit fluid ingestion at frequent intervals along the course.

It was not until 1996 that the ACSM issued a position that recommended carbohydrates be ingested during competition at a rate of 120 to 240 calories per hour to delay fatigue.

From 1975 to 1995, the emphasis on fluid intake was one of avoiding dehydration and heat disorders. For the past 20 years, the emphasis has shifted to optimizing performance by replacing calories during any endurance event exceeding 1 to 2 hours.

Now the warnings are focused on the effects of drinking too much. More deaths have come from hyponatremia than from heat disorders in road racing during the past 10 years.

I learned through experimentation that when I took water during the marathon, I was able to avoid dehydration and hyperthermia. Similarly, I discovered that by taking sports drinks and consuming carbohydrates during the marathon, I was able to avoid late-race vomiting due to my glycogen-depleted liver.

Enhancing Performance

For a while now, carbohydrates have been vilified. It started with the high-protein diet developed by Atkins and has reached a peak with the Paleo craze and the antigluten movement. But in fact, carbohydrates are the body's preferred energy source for muscle contraction. After a carbohydrate is eaten, it is broken down into smaller units of sugar, including glucose. If the body does not need that glucose for energy, it gets stored in the liver and the skeletal muscles in a form called glycogen. The stored glycogen can provide about 2,000 calories' worth of energy during a race.[1]

Glucose from muscle and liver glycogen and fatty acids released from fat stores are the two main sources for energy production in muscles. High-intensity exercise is fueled primarily by glucose, and low to moderate exercise is fueled by fat.[2] When a runner exhausts her glycogen supply, she will "hit the wall." If you have been there, you know that this is a place you never want to go, where it can take Herculean effort even to walk to the finish line.

For performance enhancement, marathon runners need to raise their lactate threshold—the pace at which carbohydrate becomes the primary source of energy—so that they can increase their capacity for fat utilization, thus saving glycogen for use later in a race. That is why good training programs include workouts designed to raise the lactate threshold, such as tempo runs that are run at the appropriate intensity.

Once we understand that the total amount of stored carbohydrate in the form of glycogen is limited and not sufficient to enable us to maintain high intensity for more than 90 to 120 minutes, we must develop strategies for sparing glycogen. These strategies should include (1) running at a pace that will increase fat use by not exceeding the lactate threshold, (2) maximizing the ability to store liver and muscle glycogen before exercise, and (3) increasing the capacity to absorb carbohydrate during exercise.[3]

In Chapter 8, we discussed the importance of pacing in detail. Now you understand why these strategies are essential. Run too fast early in a race and deplete the stored carbohydrate (glycogen) as an energy source, and your pace will suffer later in the race. So how do you pack your glycogen storage space?

Fueling Plan for the Week Prior to the Event

Carbohydrate loading is designed to increase the glycogen content in both the liver and muscles to delay the onset of fatigue. The fundamental element of the technique is to switch from a normal balanced diet to one very high in carbohydrate content.[4] The technique is recommended for endurance events lasting 90 minutes or longer.

The original, classic carbohydrate-loading technique developed by Scandinavian researchers in the early days of the boom in marathoning involved a glycogen depletion run followed by 2 to 3 days of a diet composed primarily of fats and protein and very little carbohydrate. The researchers instructed their subjects to continue with regular running.[5] Following the 3-day depletion stage, the loading began with 70 percent or more of the calories to be contributed by carbohydrates. Runners found the method effective, but it was a miserable experience because of the overall fatigue and muscular weakness associated with the depletion phase of the technique.

Current research suggests that simply changing to a very high carbohydrate diet 3 days prior to a marathon along with a taper of activity can supercompensate glycogen storage.[6] The additional glycogen storage does not enable the runner to run faster, but it does allow him to maintain a given pace longer. Most marathoners find it difficult to maintain their target paces after 2 hours. Having fuel available for the last 6 miles may prevent the nearly universal slowing most marathoners experience.

However, before you sit down to binge on pasta and bread, be aware that following a carbohydrate-rich diet 3 days prior to the endurance event does not mean eating a lot more food and calories than normal. Making any significant dietary modifications before a competition is always risky. It is important not to shock your digestive and gastrointestinal (GI) tract. Runners fear GI distress as much as they do running out of fuel.

I prefer consuming slightly more calories and a larger meal 2 days prior to the marathon, so that on the day before the marathon my total food consumption is going to be as normal as possible. I want to be confident the morning of the marathon that my GI tract is functioning normally.

Researcher Melvin H. Williams, PhD, suggests that the last large meal should occur 15 hours prior to the race.[7] I try to take the pre-race-day meal no more than 12 hours before the start of the race. You should experiment in your training runs to determine what works best.

Fueling Plan Immediately before the Event

So how much should you eat before a marathon? Williams recommends 16 to 20 calories of carbohydrate per kilogram of body weight 4 hours prior to the event.[8] For a 120-pound person, that would mean consuming 850 to 1,100 calories; for a 150-pound person, 1,100 to 1,350 calories.

However, at FIRST, we do not feel that many calories are necessary. Instead, we recommend multiplying the hours before the race times the body weight in pounds to determine the number of calories to consume.[9] For example, 4 hours before the event, a 120-pound person would consume 480 calories; a 150-pound person, 600 calories. We also recommend taking in another 100 to 150 calories (16 to 24 ounces) of sports drink 1 to 2 hours prior to the race.

As you can see in the examples above, there is a considerable discrepancy in the two recommendations. Runners vary greatly in the number of calories they normally consume just hours before a race. Some runners are accustomed to having a regular meal 3 to

4 hours before a marathon, whereas others are reluctant to eat any solid food for fear of an upset stomach. The calories can be consumed as fluids or solid food.

Many runners develop rituals and patterns (and sometimes superstitions—runners are not above magical thinking) that become part of their prerace practice. They wear the same shirt. They have a lucky drink. And they eat exactly the same food. This can be a good thing. Your prerace plan should not include anything new. Your experimentation with what best fuels your long runs adequately without causing GI issues should occur during your training. Your prerace fueling should be routine by the time of the race. You have to find what works for you.

Some elite runners swear by a banana and peanut butter. Some eat Pop-Tarts. Some just have energy gels. Other common premarathon fueling foods include oatmeal, bagels, toast, and energy bars. Some runners prefer to consume mostly liquid calories.

Before my marathons, I down an 8-ounce can of a meal supplement (Ensure, Boost) that provides 220 calories and 32 grams of carbohydrate. If you are worried about belly bloat, two cans of meal supplement can give you 440 calories with only 16 ounces of liquid. The calorie-dense supplemental meal does not inhibit gastric emptying, so you will not have a heavy feeling in your stomach.

I prefer eating 3 to 4 hours before a marathon. I want to make sure I have consumed enough calories to be prepared for the multihour event. I also want to make sure that I have eaten early enough to ensure elimination. No one wants to need a pit stop on the course.

Fueling during a Race

During a race lasting more than 90 minutes, the American College of Sports Medicine recommends that you consume 120 to 240 calories of carbohydrate every hour. If you drink 8 ounces of sports drink (14 grams of carbohydrate) every 20 minutes, you will consume 42 grams per hour, or 168 calories. Over 3 hours in a race, you will have consumed 504 calories, which will contribute to the available energy for your last few miles. It does not sound like much, but with proper pacing, it will help you avoid hitting the wall.

Whatever your preference is for consuming calories during the long endurance event, you need to have practiced that regimen during training. Remember, nothing new on race day (including shoes or shirts).

Hydration

Both too much and too little fluid can be dangerous. Dehydration can contribute to heat disorders, which will slow you down. Over-hydration can cause hyponatremia, which is a condition of a low concentration of sodium in the blood, which can slow you down and even kill you.

In his book *Waterlogged: The Serious Problem of Overhydration in Endurance Sports,* Tim Noakes, MD, exposed the danger of too much fluid ingestion.[10] Even though death from heat disorders and hyponatremia are rare, there have been more deaths from the latter than the former in the past 10 years. Dr. Noakes criticizes the sports drink industry for promoting unhealthy hydration practices.

Because individuals sweat at different rates, experience varying levels of GI discomfort, run at different paces, and come in a variety of sizes and shapes, each of us has different fluid needs. The same holds true for fluid replacement during the race. Environmental conditions also influence how much you need to drink. For that reason, the recommendation to drink when you are thirsty makes sense. That said, under normal conditions the general recommendation is to consume 8 ounces of fluid that contains small amounts of electrolytes every 20 minutes during competition.[11]

Today, you often see runners carrying water bottles and constantly drinking. (Some of my students come to class armed with enough fluid to keep them hydrated for days.) Many runners wear a fuel belt with multiple bottles even for relatively short runs or in races where there are aid stations every 2 miles. These unnecessary practices contribute to the need for so many portable restrooms.

Postrace Replenishment

During the 2 to 3 hours after the race, make sure to consume enough fluid to replace your body-weight losses. Replenish with some carbohydrate, protein, and salt in your postrace refueling.

Unfortunately, alcoholic drinks have been found to delay the recovery process.[12] So if you have just spent 26.2 miles fantasizing about beer and pizza, have some sports drink before you celebrate.

Supplementation and Ergogenic Aids

Dietary supplements advertised as performance enhancing are referred to as ergogenic aids. These sports nutrition supplements are very popular with runners. Runners are always searching for a magical food or substance. Most dietary supplements are not effective as ergogenic aids, and some are unsafe or illegal.

Nutrition supplements receive very little governmental oversight. Retailers and manufacturers have great freedom in making marketing claims.[13]

Dietary supplements vary greatly in quality. Some may contain more or less of a listed substance, and some may contain ingredients that are not listed on the label. Supplements that are mislabeled may contain substances that are harmful, such as ephedrine.[14] Supplements may provide a false sense of security for those using them as a substitute for a healthy diet. In fact, taking large doses of single nutrients and vitamins may have detrimental effects on health.[15]

Quite a few studies show that caffeine increases endurance capacity and decreases the perceived level of exertion. Caffeine has been studied extensively, and there are numerous suggested mechanisms by which caffeine provides an ergogenic effect.[16] Typically, many runners consume coffee prior to a race as part of their daily routine because it can facilitate prerace elimination, and they believe it will help their performance. Many of the gels contain caffeine in addition to carbohydrate. I believe that caffeine is beneficial. I begin my race-morning preparation with tea and coffee.

Healthy-Eating Guidelines

For public health professionals, every 5 years the federal government publishes dietary guidelines that reflect the current body of nutrition science. These recommendations are developed to help Americans make healthy food and beverage choices and to serve as the foundation for vital nutrition policies and programs across the United States. Go to health.gov/dietaryguidelines for the latest (2015) recommendations.[17]

In 2001, Walter C. Willett, MD, published *Eat, Drink, and Be Healthy: The Harvard Medical School Guide to Healthy Eating* as part of an effective campaign to discredit the USDA's familiar food pyramid. Willett exposed how agribusiness lobbying, not scientific data, drove its design.[18]

The USDA toppled the Food Guide Pyramid in 2005 and replaced it with MyPyramid—basically the old pyramid turned on its side without any explanatory text. This iteration was criticized for being vague and confusing. In June 2011, the USDA replaced MyPyramid with a new simpler food icon, the fruit-and-vegetable-rich MyPlate.[19] The Harvard School of Public Health built on MyPlate to create its Healthy Eating Plate, which takes into consideration, and puts into perspective, the wealth of

UP CLOSE AND PERSONAL

At age 50, Alan began running as part of an effort to pursue a healthier lifestyle and lose some excess weight. After shedding a few pounds, he began running 5-Ks. He admits that he had no idea about how to train. He searched for information in running books and was convinced that those books were written for former high school and college athletes, not thin-haired, overweight, lethargic, middle-aged men.

Name: Alan Newkirk
Age: 62
Hometown: Mt. Sterling, KY
Occupation: President, Total Hearth & Grill, Inc.
Race times: Marathon, 3:38 (PR) at age 61
Age he began running: 50

He picked up a copy of *Runner's World Run Less, Run Faster* at the local bookstore and began wondering if he could possibly run a marathon after he turned 60 years old. At age 59, he decided to attend a FIRST running retreat to find out if he had the potential to run a marathon.

Here is how Alan describes his running journey that took a significant turn at the FIRST retreat he attended in 2014.

- For the first time, I experienced track intervals, tempo runs, stretching, cross-training, swimming workouts, nutrition classes, form analysis, and a host of other experiences.

research conducted during the last 20 years that has reshaped the definition of healthy eating.[20]

It is likely that the recommendations will continue to change and evolve, but I find Dr. Willett's simple nutritional strategy a good basis for a healthy-eating plan.

❱ Maintain a stable, healthy weight.

❱ Replace saturated and trans fats with unsaturated fats.

❱ Substitute whole-grain carbohydrates for refined-grain carbohydrates.

- I began to believe that it would be realistic for me to train for a marathon.
- The advice and encouragement that I received from the FIRST coaches invigorated me.
- The nutritional information led me to better eating habits and enhanced my training and how I felt in general.
- The training plan that I received did not seem overwhelming.
- I followed my training plan religiously for the next 9 months.
- My wife and I traveled to Greece, where I completed my first marathon 2 weeks after I turned 60.
- Marathon running changed the entire trajectory of my life.

We are heartened by Alan's success. After his inaugural marathon in Greece, he became a marathoning Forrest Gump. He has now completed 21 marathons, including a qualifying race for the Boston Marathon, which he plans to run in 2017. He is well on his way toward his goal of running marathons on all seven continents and in all 50 states.

Alan's example shows that it is never too late to begin your running quest. His adoption of a structured plan and improved dietary habits enabled him to get fitter, faster, and healthier. His quest was enhanced because his wife, Joann, quickly became an active participant in his training and is now running half-marathons herself.

) Choose healthier sources of proteins by trading red meat for nuts, beans, chicken, and fish.

) Eat plenty of vegetables and fruits.

) Use alcohol in moderation.[21]

Or you could follow Michael Pollan's even simpler guidelines: Eat real food. Not too much. Mostly plants.[22]

Weight Management

Achieving an ideal body weight is a key factor for being healthy, fit, and, yes, fast.

At this point, even though the consequences of being overweight are widely known, more than two-thirds of Americans are overweight or obese and more than one-third are obese.

Dr. Willett boldly claimed that other than smoking, your weight is the most important measure of your future health. Further, he stated that how much you weigh in relation to your height, your waist size, and how much weight you gain after your early twenties strongly influence your chances of a host of bad outcomes. If you weigh too much, you are more likely to experience a heart attack or stroke; develop cardiovascular disease, high blood pressure, high cholesterol, or diabetes; be diagnosed with postmenopausal breast cancer or cancer of the endometrium, colon, or kidney; have arthritis; become infertile; develop gallstones; snore or suffer from sleep apnea; or develop adult-onset asthma.[23] That statement should persuade everyone to make efforts to achieve a healthy weight.

Runners generally do not think much about their weight. They persist in the belief that just by getting out the door, they are doing enough to stave off illness and pudge. At FIRST, we see how disciplined, dedicated, and determined runners are. Their goals are of utmost importance, yet we are continually perplexed by how they undermine their good efforts with excess body fat. The discipline to pull on the running shoes at 4:00 a.m.; withstand cold, heat, rain, or snow; and devote a significant portion of any free time to training is somehow not enough to resist the habit of overindulging in tasty pleasures. Of course, we realize that our culture gives us incredible access to food. Our collective willpower is constantly being tested.

The fact is, running performance is influenced by body weight. If you do not believe this, think about how much dickering goes on over the weight racehorses will carry. If 3 pounds on a half-ton horse running less than a mile make that big a difference, think about what 20 pounds on a 180-pound man over 26.2 miles will do. In a nutshell: Being overweight will slow your race times. If you want to get faster, then reduce excess body fat and get down to your optimal body weight.

Being too thin will also impair performance. Most elite runners are 10 to 20 percent below standard healthy weight ranges with very low body fat percentages. Not everyone is meant to be a lightweight, elite runner. Attempts to be ultrathin can lead to disordered eating. Unfortunately, that condition is far too common among runners, especially females.

Runners need to eat enough calories to support their training. Without proper fueling, training and racing will suffer. We encourage runners not to "diet" but to develop healthy eating plans based on sound nutritional principles. Dieting is often thought of as a temporary state to achieve a target weight for a specific event. In reality, however, it is the development of a healthy, *lifelong* eating plan that increases the likelihood of achieving your potential as a runner and decreases the likelihood of a lifestyle-related disease.

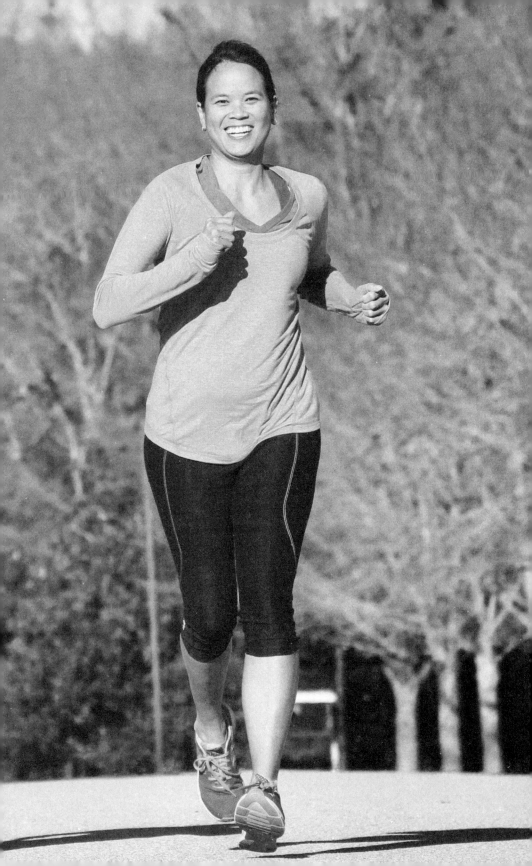

CHAPTER 10

DON'T FORGET WHY YOU ARE DOING THIS

COLLEAGUES OFTEN TELL ME THEY admire my disciplined exercise. My exercise, however, is not disciplined behavior following guidelines for healthy living. I am just doing what I enjoy. The late George Sheehan, MD, cardiologist and author, wrote that "a man's exercise must be play, or it will do him little good. Exercise that is drudgery is worthless."[1] For many years, when asked why I run, I have explained that it is my play. It is the recess that I looked forward to in elementary school.

As a physical and health educator, I realized long ago that the best counseling I can provide is to help individuals discover the physical activity that they enjoy—because that is the one they are likely to do. I try to achieve the same when coaching runners. I strive to design a training program that will help them achieve their goals and that they will also enjoy.

Roger Bannister, the first man to break the 4-minute-mile barrier, wrote, "My ideal athlete was first and foremost a human being who ran his sport and did not allow it to run him."[2] I have observed too many runners who miss the joy of running by letting it become one more stressor in their lives. Training becomes drudgery. Finish times become disappointments. Training interferes with relationships and disrupts family life. But I believe running need not become one more obligation.

When I was a college basketball coach, I told my players that the most important lesson they could learn was to know themselves. Self-examination is crucial on the road to self-discovery. They would perform better knowing their strengths and weaknesses. The team would perform better if the players collectively recognized their strengths and weaknesses.

The same self-knowledge is true for runners. Know what type of training you find effective and enjoyable. If you prefer 10-Ks, do not run marathons just because others in your running group or club are doing so.

The Joy of Running

Roger Bannister writes, "It will be difficult to describe how moments when running seems utterly insignificant alternate with moments when it threatens to engulf me."[3] Dr. Sheehan similarly writes, "In play, you realize simultaneously the supreme importance and utter insignificance of what you are doing."[4] The Dutch historian Johan Huizinga stated that performing an activity with utmost seriousness with the results inconsequential was the essence of play.[5]

Bannister points out there are times when we are totally focused on our running performances. It can consume our thoughts and behavior. Yet when we step back and examine our stressing over race finish times of a few seconds or minutes, we recognize our preoccupation as irrational and meaningless in the larger scheme of life.

The key to making your running a joyful, meaningful activity devoid of stress, obsession, and depression is being able to immerse yourself in the activity without experiencing any stressful residue once you've completed the run. Rachel Toor writes, "Away from the exigencies of daily life, you are free not to think about them. And so, often, you don't."[6] Let your running be that escape from daily stressors.

Dr. Sheehan also writes that "joy comes at the peak of an experience."[7] That fits with Huizinga's description of play as something done with utmost seriousness. I agree that joy, satisfaction, and even a physical euphoria can accompany an intense effort. Learning to enjoy that hard effort without being overly concerned with the numbers on the watch is one of the keys to achieving and maintaining a healthy and joyful running habit.

It is always good to have a challenge, even a minor one. Pick a goal that challenges you. Do not let it be something potentially harmful. At the same time, remember that determination and a goal can become a disease if not kept in proper perspective.

Leave room in your training for spontaneity. Sakyong Mipham, author of *Running with the Mind of Meditation,* declared that spontaneity can serve to reawaken and bring energy into what you are doing.[8]

Relive Childhood: Run Fast Sometimes

Watch children run. They race across the yard, stop, recover, and take off again. They definitely experience intensity. I wonder if our infatuation with marathons and even ultramarathons has not led to a loss of the zestful, youthful experience associated with intensity. I feel most youthful when I am doing intervals or even pushing hard on a fast tempo run. That is why I advocate that runners not forsake the shorter races.

The FIRST training programs in *Runner's World Run Less, Run Faster* use a 5-K time for determining target training paces. Runners often tell us that they have not run a race shorter than a half- or full marathon in years. They will not only benefit by becoming faster runners through training for and racing 5-Ks, 8-Ks, and 10-Ks but will also experience the intensity that elicits a youthful sensation.

Keep It Fresh and Balanced

As Amby Burfoot, winner of the 1968 Boston Marathon and the former executive editor of *Runner's World*, writes in *The Runner's Guide to the Meaning of Life*, "Starting lines are one of the most important stations of life. We need to do more than just avoid them. We need to actively seek them out. Otherwise, we grow stagnant. We will disappear into black holes."[9] He adds, "A run is most meaningful and most enjoyable when it exists for its own sake, when it doesn't feel the pressure of a ticking stopwatch."[10]

Burfoot recognizes the value of seeking new challenges and also enjoying the activity itself. Establishing a goal, training for it, and entering a race while enjoying our training and racing require a balance that we should all strive to achieve. Burfoot is a model for us all. Over more than 50 years, he has demonstrated the pure joy of running interspersed with periodic racing goals. Through his prolific writing, he has taught runners how to strive for excellence and keep running as a pleasurable activity.

Running Is a Special Competition: Embrace It

Years ago, I was fortunate to be out front in local races and experience the cheers of the crowd, much like being applauded during my basketball career. What I learned about running is that the spectators' shouts of encouragement were just as loud when I was more than an hour behind the leaders. Running is different from other sports in that the observers root for everyone. Those who have run the Boston Marathon know that the cheers are deafening as you go through Framingham and especially through Wellesley—where college students make a scream tunnel—no matter where you are among the 30,000 runners. That is rare in sports, where typically fans pull only for their teams.

The same egalitarian spirit holds true for how runners treat one another. You can race someone with every ounce of energy you have all the way to the finish line, and regardless of which one of you wins, you immediately shake hands or embrace each other for having shared the common experience. That does not happen in other sports, or if it does, it is done out of courtesy or adherence to socially acceptable protocol. In running, the spirit is genuine.

The positive support provided by runners and running spectators is one of the reasons that I enjoy the sport. How many times when you were struggling in a race has a fellow runner come by and encouraged you by offering to stick with you to the finish line? Or passed you and said, "Good job"?

Be Smart with Your Racing

We began this book by saying our purpose in writing is to help runners make running a healthy, lifelong activity. That requires being smart about your racing. Let races become your playground, not your proving ground.

Overall, we believe there is too much marathoning. While some runners can handle high-mileage training year after year, most encounter injuries. Runners need to properly prepare for a marathon and properly recover from the event. Limit your marathoning to one per year in most years. Occasionally doing two is okay.

We also find that many runners race once or twice per month. When is there time to train if you are continually tapering and recovering for and from these races?

Pace yourself for the long run. I am not only talking about your race pace but also the number and spacing of races you enter over several years. Racing less frequently makes your races more special.

Stay Injury-Free

Remember, the best predictor of an injury is having had a previous injury. Therefore, you want to prevent the initial injury. The problem is that uninjured runners will not think that the advice for moderation we are offering in this book applies to them.

Take time off periodically to fully recover. You are especially vulnerable after a marathon, even if you feel completely recovered.

Do not feel compelled to continue training for your next race when you are injured. Get well and start planning for another race in your future. Many of the questions we receive at FIRST pertain to how runners can manage their training with an injury with only a given number of weeks to go before the race. It's common for us to receive a message from a runner asking which of the following options he should choose.

Skip the track repeats and do just the tempo and long run?

Cut back on the pace and do all three workouts?

Take a week off completely and then resume training?

Do cross-training for key runs #1 and #2 and do the long run?

UP CLOSE AND PERSONAL

W e could not provide you with a better example of how to put it all together to be fit, fast, and healthy. Brian has incorporated all the smart training principles into his weekly training regimen.

Name: Brian Joel

Age: 61

Occupation: CEO/President, POSitec Solutions Inc.

Hometown: Surrey, BC, Canada

Race times: 10-K, 44:54; half-marathon, 1:41:43; marathon, 3:44:11

Age he began running: 50

Brian was active in his youth. At age 39, he started his own business, which he built into a multimillion-dollar operation. But that came with a cost. The long hours he spent developing the business brought stress and poor eating habits and left no time for exercise. When he hit 50, his doctor told him that he needed a change in lifestyle.

Brian started running and set a goal of getting into better shape and developing a better-quality life. To keep the running motivating, he signed up for a few 10-Ks. He ran his first full marathon at age 52 in 4:22. With more serious training, his extra effort was causing injuries. He ran five more marathons but could not break 4 hours. The injuries persisted.

He decided he needed a new approach to his training. He began going to the gym to stretch and perform strength exercises. He reduced the number of days that he was running, but he became focused on making each run a quality workout. He further changed his dietary habits and began making healthy eating choices. He replaced a couple run workouts with cycling.

All of these changes led to a 3:44 marathon, which reinforced his adoption of his new training regimen.

At 60, Brian had completely changed his lifestyle and reported that he slept better, dealt with stress better, and felt more energetic. He also indicated that he had influenced his entire family to adopt healthier behaviors.

Brian's doctor, impressed with his transformation, told him, "Please don't stop running."

At FIRST, we are health educators as well as exercise scientists, so preaching the message of wellness and balance comes as naturally to us as coaching runners to go faster. Brian represents what we hope to accomplish with this book—promoting lifelong running as a healthy, fun activity.

Typically following the options is the statement *Not running this race is not an option.*

Every runner at some time will face the decision of not racing, even after months of preparation and invested travel expenses. It takes courage to interrupt training and revise goals—those people who do so are the smart runners. The runners who ignore their bodies and run when their injury is serious enough to interrupt their training will in most cases have a disappointing race finish and exacerbate their injuries, which often means making the next race they hoped to run questionable. I cannot count the number of times I've observed this scenario. I have watched runners limp along, continuing to race year after year, until they can no longer run. And not being able to run can have serious health consequences. Once you become inactive, the beneficial aspects associated with aerobic physical activity are lost. Weight and waist size increase. Cholesterol and triglycerides increase. You lose stamina and muscle mass.

Mipham writes that the wise are balanced and the foolish are extreme.[11] All of us go through periods when we are foolish with our training and racing, he says. Running longevity requires wisdom. Respect your injuries, and use this handbook to become a balanced and lifelong runner so you can maintain the health benefits associated with running and longevity.

Running Benefits Extend beyond Fast Times and Good Health

"I hoped my striving as an athlete would liberate other potentialities which I knew existed inside me," Roger Bannister writes.[12] He adds, "It also does us good because it helps us do other things better."[13]

Runners develop discipline in their lives because the training regimen requires it. That disciplined behavior often transfers to work, diet, and even hobbies. As college professors, we observe that cross-country runners are typically excellent students even though they train vigorously once or twice per day. They learn the benefits of having good habits.

Running contributes to enhanced self-esteem. That's because conscientious efforts in running yield positive results. This is not true of all athletic disciplines, as I've learned from teaching and coaching other sports. Because many sports require a certain degree of coordination, quickness, balance, or speed, some individuals see little development from their efforts. I like to coach runners because I can guarantee success if they adhere to their training program.

Confidence arises in the body through physical movement and in the mind through gaining knowledge, Mipham writes.[14] I have observed high school and college students become more confident individuals as a result of experiencing improvement as runners.

Running and Friendship

"Running with another person is an intimate activity," Rachel Toor says. "Run with someone long enough at a time and you will be stripped bare. Modesty falls away with the miles. The body—its functions, its excretions, its wants—cannot be ignored. The heavy breathing, the sweating, the soft talk that comes after exertion, the hours spent together—the running with another person is an intimate activity. It's hard to keep the heart uninvolved."[15]

What is it that causes runners to share intimate details about their lives with their running mates? I have heard about romantic anguish, divorces, problem children, contentious teens, the death of parents, hated bosses, excitement over a new love, great jobs, children's accomplishments, and wonderful vacations.

People are more honest with their feelings in running conversations, Mipham notes. He postulates that the free and spirited expression may come about because we are in motion. Inhaling and exhaling relaxes our uptight and conceptual mind and our social persona.[16]

Does running release inhibitions and remove the barriers that prevent more personal conversations? My experiences confirm the notion that running with another person lessens one's self-consciousness and leads to more open exchanges.

In the past, I taught a first-year seminar that focused on the philosophical, psychological, and sociological aspects of running. The students read Rachel Toor's book *Personal Record,* which includes the quote that opened this section. One topic explored throughout the semester was why runners will talk more freely with someone while running than when sitting together having a conversation. The consensus was that it is easier to talk when not looking directly at someone's face.

This intimacy among runners appears to be widespread. In my classes, I always bring in a panel of female runners, who vary in age from thirties to sixties, to discuss what they like about running. Tops on their lists are the close bonds and personal conversations. The panelists often state that their closest friends are fellow runners with whom they can share the most confidential parts of their lives.

If happiness is the ability to share what we have with others, then running becomes a catalyst for happiness. The secret to long-term happiness is engaging in activities that are healthy—mentally and physically.

How to Find the Right Balance

Running can add zest to your life. But like salt applied to food, too much of it can ruin the taste; too little of it fails to enhance. The key is to balance frequency, intensity, duration, and, most important, perspective. You need the right dose of running for performance success and to avoid injury. You need the right level of importance placed on your running to keep it playful, joyful, and fun. That balance is different for each individual. Finding your balance is essential to your becoming a healthy, fit, fast, and joyful lifelong runner.

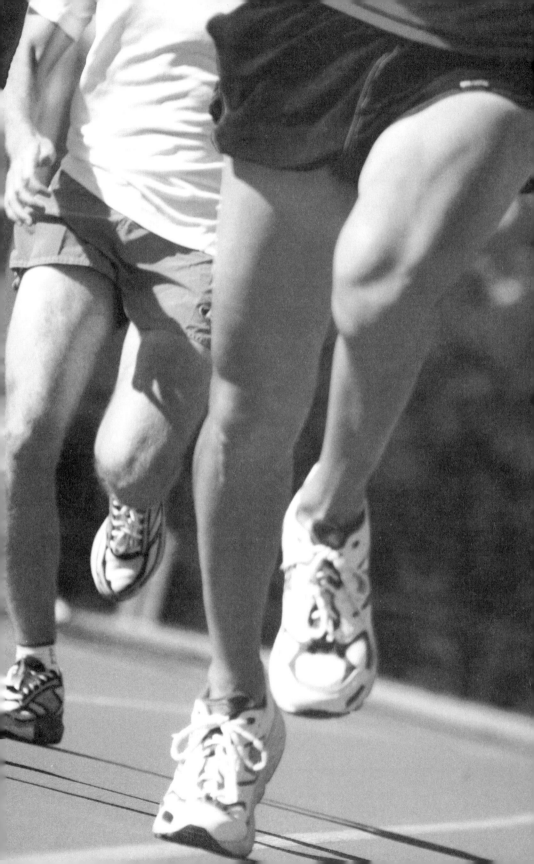

THE PLAN

PUTTING IT ALL TOGETHER

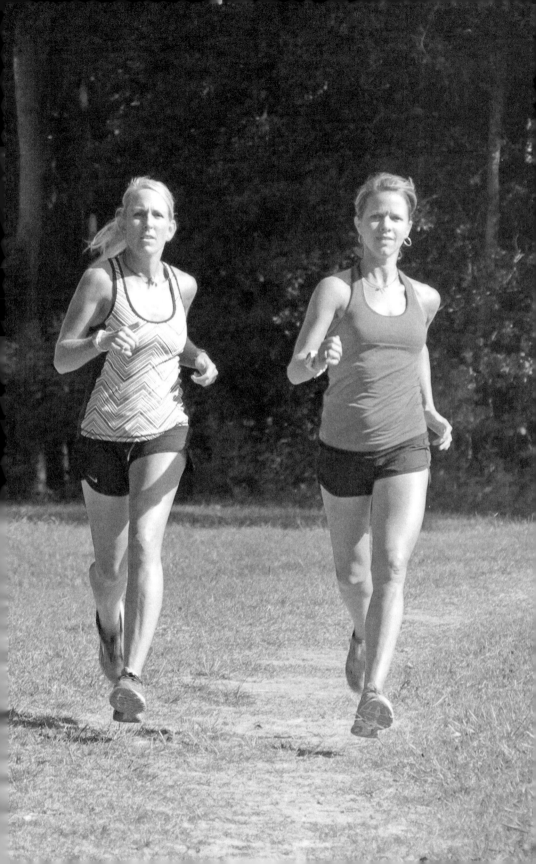

CHAPTER 11

THE 7-HOUR WORKOUT WEEK

CAN I TRAIN SMART TO become a lifelong runner? Do I have enough time in my busy week to develop, improve, and maintain a high level of fitness? Can I become fit without spending a fortune on expensive equipment and memberships? At FIRST, we believe the answer to all of these questions is yes.

Based on our experiences as lifelong runners, coaches, and exercise scientists, we have developed the 7-Hour Workout Week. The 7 hours include activities to enhance cardiorespiratory endurance, muscular strength and endurance, and flexibility. While we have access to sophisticated training and analytic equipment, we have found that our own training for lifelong fitness is done with minimal equipment—a physio ball, a stretching mat, a few dumbbells, and some stretch bands.

Our 7-Hour Workout Week is designed to develop overall fitness and running speed while reducing the likelihood of injury. The schedule was developed to enable runners to use it for lifelong running as well as for race preparation for 5-Ks,

10-Ks, and half-marathons. It is designed for general fitness and health enhancement, even when there is no targeted future race.

The 7-Hour Workout Week is an ideal base for beginning a marathon training program. Actually, with minor modifications, such as adding a few longer runs, it could serve well for marathon training.

Why 7 hours? Because most of the runners we come across have busy lives and cannot devote more time to training. As we have written throughout this book, our goal is to help you achieve optimal benefits with limited training. For us, the daily hour is generally at lunchtime. While 7 hours per week mean an average of an hour of training each day, this training schedule will enable you to achieve a high level of physical fitness, be prepared to race, and develop a plan for becoming a lifelong, healthy runner.

Yes, you might become fitter and maybe faster by doing more, but in the process you'd risk injury and/or burnout while creating an imbalance with other priorities in your life. This plan aims to create a healthy balance among work, family, and other outside interests and pursuits even as it sets serious running goals.

The 7-Hour Workout Week activities provide variety and address all the determinants of running performance and the components of physical fitness. Detailed descriptions of how to perform the plan's strength and flexibility exercises are found in Chapters 12 and 13.

We learned from runners responding to both editions of *Run Less, Run Faster* that runners like specific workouts. "Just tell me what to do and I will do it" is one of the most common phrases we hear from runners. That's why we provide a prescriptive workout for each day of the week.

As we developed the 7-Hour Workout Week, we asked ourselves if each workout could easily be done. That is, we want to make sure that the workouts are not too difficult to perform, that they do not require a specific facility, and that they involve only minimal equipment. No matter how good an exercise or workout plan is, if it isn't something you're likely to follow, the plan will not produce the desired outcome.

We perform these exercises. We know how long it takes to complete them. The benefits from doing the strength exercises, stretches, and cross-training are significant for runners.

Many runners have confessed to us that they skip the recommended resistance training, stretching, and cross-training. Yes, runners like to run, just run. But to become healthy, fit, and fast requires more than just running. Give the weekly plan a chance to help you become a lifelong runner.

Before we get into the day-by-day plan, let's begin with a brief description of each element.

Run Workouts

The three run workouts of the 7-Hour Workout Week are the same three types of runs included in the FIRST training programs. We have documented the success of thousands of runners using those key run workouts. In the 7-Hour Workout Week, we focus on time and intensity of effort for each run rather than on pace and distance as in *Run Less, Run Faster*.

Each run workout is designed to effect improvement in one or more of the performance determinants: aerobic capacity, lactate threshold, running economy, and running speed.

For lifelong running, you need to know what reinforces your running and what causes stress—physical or mental. If having a target pace in minutes and seconds for every run creates mental stress and takes away enjoyment, you will eventually find an excuse not to continue with the activity, especially if you began running for the pure joy of it.

If having a challenging target pace for each run causes you physical stress that leads to repeated injuries, that may ultimately become a reason to discontinue what otherwise had been an enjoyable activity. For those who prefer to rely on how they feel rather than on the numbers on a watch, we designate intensities using the FIRST Exertion Scale (FES) found on pages 153–154.

For those runners more accustomed to assessing their workout intensity based on pace and time targets, Appendix A displays a handy table that provides the pace per mile and pace per kilometer equivalents to the perceived exertion levels from the FES that can be used for the 7-Hour Workout Week run workouts. We realize that many runners now rely on their GPS with the current pace displayed for monitoring their workout intensity.

For those who would like to incorporate additional variety into their workouts, Appendix B details supplemental run workouts that you can swap out.

Our goal is to forge a training program that enables you to be fit and healthy. The FES serves as a good tool for ensuring that you get the stimulus necessary for the physical adaptations that lead to maintaining and improving your fitness level.

Cross-Training Is Smart Training for Lifelong Running

Running, cycling, strength training, core work, yoga, and numerous other options are great forms of exercise. Each can improve aspects of your fitness. Which ones do you need? Do you need to do all of them?

Many runners adopt a training schedule and change just the distances that they run. If they run a PR in a race, they might repeat a training program over and over. To maintain effective workouts over the long term, cross-training with variety can challenge both your muscular fitness and your cardiovascular fitness. Those varied exercises force your body to adapt to each new stimulus. Adopting a well-balanced program for improving fitness will help you avoid a plateau in your fitness efforts.

Whether you run, bike, or use an elliptical trainer, your heart does not know the difference. It only knows it has to work harder when you exercise. Cardio cross-training strengthens your heart and improves aerobic fitness. Different modes of aerobic exercise can remove the significant impact running places on the legs.

Keep your body ready to deal with novelty. Make each workout different from the previous one. There are literally thousands of different exercises that the human body can perform. The key is to make your body *adapt* to new stimuli as often as possible.

Here are a few reasons why you want to add cross-training to your weekly routine.

❱ Cross-training reduces the risk of overuse injuries by shifting the demand across different muscle groups. When you stress your muscles repetitively, they fatigue. You improve by stressing muscles, then permitting them to recover and adapt, so that they become stronger.

❱ Cross-training allows for a higher volume of aerobic training. Cross-training enables the runner to experience a greater training volume than doing an easy recovery run, which still fatigues the same muscles but does little to improve cardiorespiratory fitness.

❱ Cross-training may enhance muscle balance by developing opposing muscle groups more uniformly.

❱ Cross-training provides for total fitness of both the upper and lower body.

- Cross-training allows for a greater daily intensity of training, since the same muscle groups are not utilized each day.

- Cross-training helps keep caloric output high, and optimal body fat percentages can be achieved and maintained much more easily.

- Cross-training promotes an increased range of motion, thus reducing the risk of specific muscle tightness, helping to reduce the likelihood of injury.

- Cross-training enhances performance in running efficiency. A faster leg turnover and increased hip, knee, and ankle range of motion can improve running mechanics and economy of movement.

- Cross-training provides flexibility in the workout schedule. If the weather is horrible or conditions are not good for running, an indoor workout provides a training opportunity.

- Cross-training provides variety to the training regimen and forestalls boredom. This variety may enhance the desire to train and help athletes avoid staleness and overtraining.

- Cross-training promotes recovery. Through cross-training, runners contribute to their fitness while recovering between high-quality run workouts.

Things to Consider

Many runners have written us to say that cross-training enabled them to run a marathon. They say that they were never able to make it to the marathon starting line uninjured using other programs, but that by interspersing cross-training with their runs, they were able to stay healthy and injury-free.

We believe it is important for runners to choose activities that complement their running. Activities such as stationary cycling, rowing, and elliptical trainers all provide good cardiovascular benefits without additional stress on the knees. These modes of exercise are typically readily available and do not require much setup or preparation.

Cycling is recommended for aerobic cross-training because it can increase hip and knee joint flexibility. Cycling can also increase leg turnover and running speed. We recommend stationary cycling because it is an efficient use of time and permits a continuous aerobic workout.

Rowing on an "erg," such as a Concept2 rower, provides a non-weight-bearing workout that involves the large muscles. Rowing can be an intense workout and promotes total body fitness.

Cross-training on an elliptical trainer gives runners the opportunity to mimic a runninglike motion without the strenuous impact on the joints that occurs when running. Most elliptical trainers are now equipped with movable handles so that people can exercise their upper body and lower body simultaneously. And most elliptical trainers allow you to stride in reverse, which can activate different muscle groups.

FIRST Exertion Scale (FES)

The FES is used to gauge the intensity of exercise. The scale runs from 1 to 10. The numbers are tied to descriptions of the effort that an activity requires.

1. Very easy and relaxed
2. Relaxed effort with a slight increase in heart rate

3. A steady aerobic effort with breathing normal

4. Aware of effort but not experiencing any difficulties

5. Not laboring but having to stay focused to maintain effort

6. Having to coax yourself to maintain intensity

7. Comfortably hard; audible breathing; conversation has ceased

8. Heavy breathing; really hard effort

9. Very heavy breathing; can sustain only for a few minutes

10. Very, very hard; maximal effort

The 7-Hour Workout Week

Monday: Cross-train 30 minutes, strength train 15 minutes, stretch 10 minutes

Tuesday: Dynamic stretch 5 minutes, run 50 minutes, stretch 10 minutes

Wednesday: Cross-train 30 minutes, strength train 15 minutes, stretch 10 minutes

Thursday: Dynamic stretch 5 minutes, run 50 minutes, stretch 10 minutes

Friday: Strength train 15 minutes, stretch 10 minutes

Saturday: Dynamic stretch 5 minutes, run 60–90 minutes, stretch 15 minutes

Sunday: Cross-train 30 minutes, stretch 10 minutes

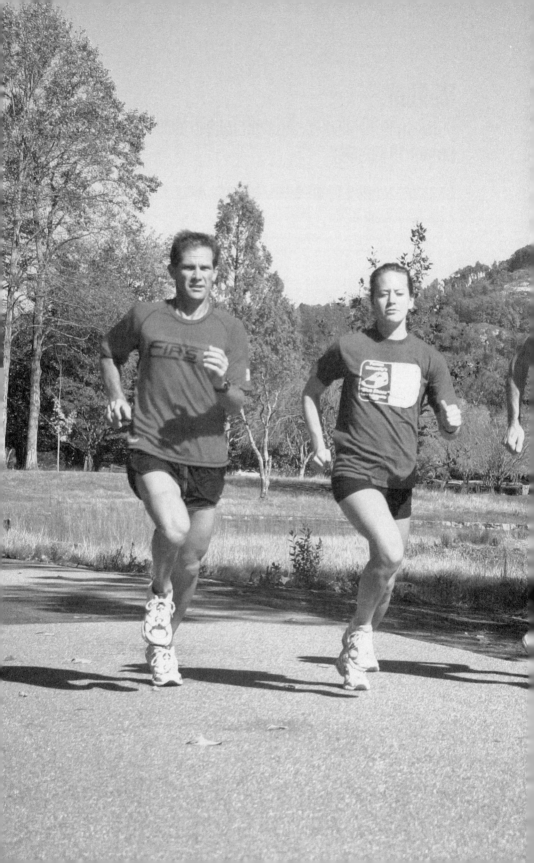

MONDAY:
Cross-Train 30 Minutes, Strength Train 15 Minutes, Stretch 10 Minutes

CROSS-TRAINING WORKOUTS (CHOOSE ONE)

Cycling Workout #1
- Begin with 5 minutes of cycling at cadence of 80+ rpm at FES of 2–3.
- 4 x (3 minutes of fast cycling [90–100 rpm] at FES of 5 followed by 2 minutes at FES of 3).
- End with 5 minutes of relaxed cycling at FES of 2 as a cooldown.

Cycling Workout #2
- Begin with 5 minutes of cycling at cadence of 80+ rpm at FES of 2–3.
- 2 x (5 minutes at FES of 5 with cadence of at least 90 rpm followed by 5 minutes at FES of 3 with cadence of 95–100 rpm).
- End with 5 minutes of relaxed cycling at FES of 2 as a cooldown.

Rowing Workout
- 5 minutes of easy rowing at FES of 2.
- 2 x (2000 meters at FES of 5 with 2-minute recovery at FES of 2).
- 2 minutes of easy rowing at FES of 2 as a cooldown.

Elliptical Workout
- 3 minutes easy at FES of 2.
- 5 x (4 minutes focused at FES of 5 with 1-minute recovery at FES of 2).
- 2 minutes easy at FES of 2 as a cooldown.

FIRST Exertion Scale (FES)

1	Very easy and relaxed
2	Relaxed effort with a slight increase in heart rate
3	A steady aerobic effort with breathing normal
4	Aware of effort but not experiencing any difficulties
5	Not laboring but having to stay focused to maintain effort
6	Having to coax yourself to maintain intensity
7	Comfortably hard; audible breathing; conversation has ceased
8	Heavy breathing; really hard effort
9	Very heavy breathing; can sustain only for a few minutes
10	Very, very hard; maximal effort

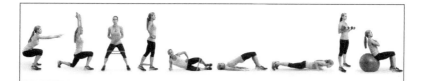

STRENGTH (RESISTANCE) EXERCISES (15 MINUTES)

(For images and information on these exercises, see Chapter 12.)

Body-Weight Squat
- 60 seconds

Walking Lunges with Hands Overhead
- 15 steps each leg

Lateral Steps with Miniband
- 15 steps each side

Kickbacks with Miniband
- 15 reps each leg

Clamshell with Miniband
- 15 reps each leg

Bridge/Pelvic Thrust with Feet Flat
- 20 reps with pause

Pushups (Standard or Modified)
- 60 seconds

Dumbbell Curl to Press
- 20 reps

Abdominal Crunch on Exercise Ball
- 60 seconds

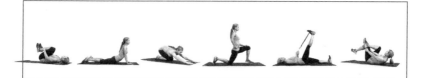

STRETCHES (10 MINUTES)

(For images and information on these stretches, see Chapter 13.)

Lower-Back Stretch #1
- 30 seconds

Cobra/Prone Back Extension
- 30 seconds

Lower-Back Stretch #2
- 30 seconds

Tall Kneeling Stretch
- 30 seconds each side

Hamstring with Rope
- 30 seconds each side

Piriformis Stretch
- 30 seconds each side

TUESDAY:
Dynamic Stretch 5 Minutes, Run 50 Minutes, Stretch 10 Minutes

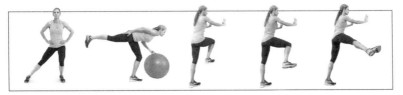

DYNAMIC STRETCHES (BEFORE RUN, 5 MINUTES)

(For images and information on these stretches, see Chapter 13.)

Dynamic Side Lunge
- 30 seconds each leg

Dynamic Single-Leg Dead Lift
- 30 seconds each leg

Dynamic Bent-Knee Forward Swing
- 12 reps each leg

Dynamic Bent-Knee Lateral Swing
- 12 reps each leg

Dynamic Straight-Leg Lateral Swing
- 12 reps each leg

RUN WORKOUTS (CHOOSE ONE)

- Begin with 15 minutes of easy running, progressing from FES of 1 to 3. Finish the workout with 5 minutes of easy running at FES of 2.
- **Run #1:** 25-minute run alternating at FES of 7–8 and FES of 3 every 5 minutes, starting with a hard effort so that you get three hard efforts of 5 minutes.
- **Run #2:** 8 x (2 minutes of fast running at FES of 9 with 60 seconds of rest recovery after each fast 2-minute interval).
- **Run #3:** 6 x (3 minutes of fast running at FES of 8 with 90 seconds of rest recovery after each fast 3-minute interval).
- **Run #4:** 4 x (5 minutes at FES of 7 with 2 minutes of rest recovery after each fast 5-minute interval).

FIRST Exertion Scale (FES)

1	Very easy and relaxed
2	Relaxed effort with a slight increase in heart rate
3	A steady aerobic effort with breathing normal
4	Aware of effort but not experiencing any difficulties
5	Not laboring but having to stay focused to maintain effort
6	Having to coax yourself to maintain intensity
7	Comfortably hard; audible breathing; conversation has ceased
8	Heavy breathing; really hard effort
9	Very heavy breathing; can sustain only for a few minutes
10	Very, very hard; maximal effort

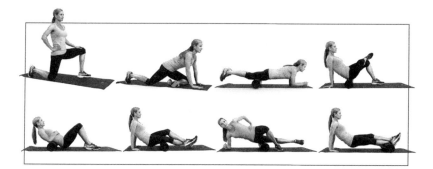

STRETCHES (AFTER RUN, 10 MINUTES)

(For images and information on these stretches, see Chapter 13.)

Open High Kneel
- 30 seconds each leg

Pigeon Pose
- 30 seconds each leg

Quadriceps with Roller
- 60 seconds

Piriformis Stretch with Roller
- 45 seconds each side

Lower Back with Roller
- 60 seconds

Hamstrings with Roller
- 45 seconds each side

ITB with Roller
- 45 seconds each side

Gastrocnemius with Roller
- 45 seconds each side

WEDNESDAY:
Cross-Train 30 Minutes, Strength Train 15 Minutes, Stretch 10 Minutes

CROSS-TRAINING WORKOUTS (CHOOSE ONE)

Cycling Workout #1
- Begin with 5 minutes of cycling at cadence of 80+ rpm at FES of 2 followed by 20-minute tempo effort at FES of 6.
- End with 5 minutes of cycling at FES of 2 as a cooldown.

Cycling Workout #2
- Begin with 5 minutes of cycling at cadence of 80+ rpm at FES of 2.
- 2 x (8 minutes at 90+ rpm at FES of 7 followed by 2 minutes at FES of 3).
- End with 5 minutes of cycling at FES of 2 as a cooldown.

Rowing Workout
- 4 minutes of rowing at FES of 3 as a warmup; rest 1 minute.
- Row 5,000 meters at FES of 7–8.
- 2 minutes of rowing at FES of 2 as a cooldown.

Elliptical Workout
- 4 minutes at FES of 3 as a warmup.
- 6 x (1 minute at FES of 4, 1 minute at FES of 5, 1 minute at FES of 7, 1 minute at FES of 2).
- 2 minutes at FES of 2 as a cooldown.

FIRST Exertion Scale (FES)

1	Very easy and relaxed
2	Relaxed effort with a slight increase in heart rate
3	A steady aerobic effort with breathing normal
4	Aware of effort but not experiencing any difficulties
5	Not laboring but having to stay focused to maintain effort
6	Having to coax yourself to maintain intensity
7	Comfortably hard; audible breathing; conversation has ceased
8	Heavy breathing; really hard effort
9	Very heavy breathing; can sustain only for a few minutes
10	Very, very hard; maximal effort

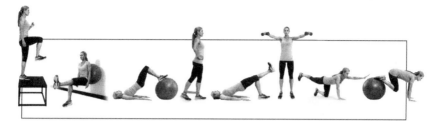

STRENGTH (RESISTANCE) EXERCISES (15 MINUTES)

(For images and information on these exercises, see Chapter 12.)

Box Stepups
- 30 seconds up and down with right foot; repeat with left foot

Single-Leg Wall Squat with Exercise Ball
- 20 reps each leg

Hip Extension Leg Curl with Exercise Ball
- 30 leg curls

Kickbacks with Miniband
- 15 reps each leg

Single-Leg Bridge/Pelvic Thrust
- 20 reps each leg with pause

Dumbbell Clocker Shoulder Raise
- 5 reps at each of the four clock positions

Quadruped/Pointer Dog
- 15 reps each side, hold each rep for 3 seconds

Reverse Crunch with Exercise Ball
- 60 seconds

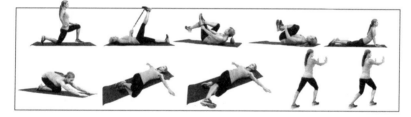

STRETCHES (10 MINUTES)

(For images and information on these stretches, see Chapter 13.)

Tall Kneeling Stretch
- 30 seconds each side

Hamstring with Rope
- 30 seconds each side

Piriformis Stretch
- 30 seconds each side

Lower-Back Stretch #1
- 30 seconds

Cobra/Prone Back Extension
- 30 seconds

Lower-Back Stretch #2
- 30 seconds

Spinal Rotation
- 30 seconds each side

Hip Abductors/ITB with Spinal Rotation
- 30 seconds each side

Isolated Gastrocnemius Stretch
- 30 seconds each leg

Isolated Soleus Stretch
- 30 seconds each leg

THURSDAY:
Dynamic stretch 5 minutes, Run 50 Minutes, Stretch 10 Minutes

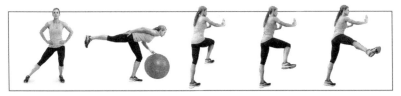

DYNAMIC STRETCHES (BEFORE RUN, 5 MINUTES)

(For images and information on these stretches, see Chapter 13.)

Dynamic Side Lunge
- 30 seconds each leg

Dynamic Single-Leg Dead Lift
- 30 seconds each leg

Dynamic Bent-Knee Forward Swing
- 12 reps each leg

Dynamic Bent-Knee Lateral Swing
- 12 reps each leg

Dynamic Straight-Leg Lateral Swing
- 12 reps each leg

RUN WORKOUTS (CHOOSE ONE)

- Begin running 15 minutes, progressing from FES of 1 to 3. Finish the workout with 5 minutes of easy running at FES of 2.
- **Run #1:** 30-minute run with focused effort at FES of 5.
- **Run #2:** 20 minutes of running at FES of 6 followed by 10 minutes of recovery running at FES of 3.
- **Run #3:** 15 minutes of running at FES of 7 followed by 5 minutes of running at FES of 3 then 10 minutes of running at FES of 7.

FIRST Exertion Scale (FES)

1	Very easy and relaxed
2	Relaxed effort with a slight increase in heart rate
3	A steady aerobic effort with breathing normal
4	Aware of effort but not experiencing any difficulties
5	Not laboring but having to stay focused to maintain effort
6	Having to coax yourself to maintain intensity
7	Comfortably hard; audible breathing; conversation has ceased
8	Heavy breathing; really hard effort
9	Very heavy breathing; can sustain only for a few minutes
10	Very, very hard; maximal effort

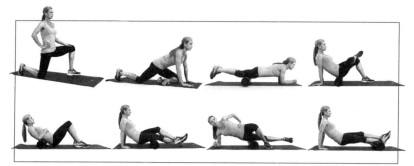

STRETCHES (AFTER RUN, 10 MINUTES)

(For images and information on these stretches, see Chapter 13.)

Open High Kneel
- 30 seconds each leg

Pigeon Pose
- 30 seconds each leg

Quadriceps with Roller
- 60 seconds

Piriformis Stretch with Roller
- 45 seconds each side

Lower Back with Roller
- 60 seconds

Hamstrings with Roller
- 45 seconds each side

ITB with Roller
- 45 seconds each side

Gastrocnemius with Roller
- 45 seconds each side

FRIDAY:
Strength Train 15 minutes, Stretch 10 minutes

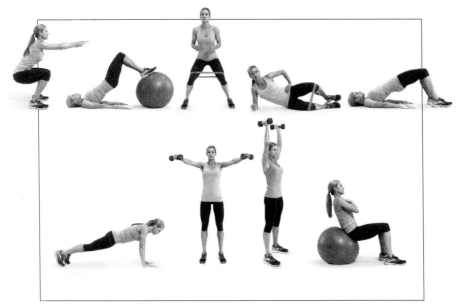

STRENGTH (RESISTANCE) EXERCISES (15 MINUTES)

(For images and information on these exercises, see Chapter 12.)

Body-Weight Squat
- 30 seconds

Hip Extension Leg Curl with Exercise Ball
- 20 leg curls

Lateral Steps with Miniband
- 15 steps each side

Clamshell with Miniband
- 15 reps each leg

Bridge/Pelvic Thrust with Feet Flat
- 20 reps with pause

Pushups (Standard or Modified)
- 30 seconds

Dumbbell Clocker Shoulder Raise
- 5 reps at each of the four clock positions

Dumbbell Curl to Press
- 20 reps

Abdominal Crunch on Exercise Ball
- 60 seconds

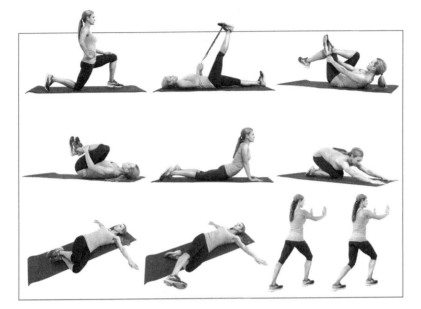

STRETCHES (10 MINUTES)

(For images and information on these stretches, see Chapter 13.)

Tall Kneeling Stretch
- 30 seconds each side

Hamstring with Rope
- 30 seconds each side

Piriformis Stretch
- 30 seconds each side

Lower-Back Stretch #1
- 30 seconds

Cobra/Prone Back Extension
- 30 seconds

Lower-Back Stretch #2
- 30 seconds

Spinal Rotation
- 30 seconds each side

Hip Abductors/ITB with Spinal Rotation
- 30 seconds each side

Isolated Gastrocnemius Stretch
- 30 seconds each leg

Isolated Soleus Stretch
- 30 seconds each leg

SATURDAY:
Dynamic Stretch 5 Minutes, Run 60–90 Minutes, Stretch 15 Minutes

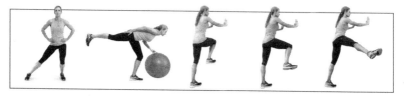

DYNAMIC STRETCHES (BEFORE RUN, 5 MINUTES)

(For images and information on these stretches, see Chapter 13.)

Dynamic Side Lunge
- 30 seconds each leg

Dynamic Single-Leg Deadlift
- 30 seconds each leg

Dynamic Bent-Knee Forward Swing
- 12 reps each leg

Dynamic Bent-Knee Lateral Swing
- 12 reps each leg

Dynamic Straight-Leg Lateral Swing
- 12 reps each leg

RUN WORKOUTS (CHOOSE ONE)

- Begin to run comfortably, progressing from 1 to 3 on the FES scale. After 10 minutes of running, gradually pick up the pace and continue as specified in each of the four runs.
- **Run #1:** Continue the run at FES of 4 for the remainder of the 60 minutes.
- **Run #2:** Continue the run at FES of 4 for 30 minutes and finish with 30 minutes at FES of 5.
- **Run #3:** Continue the run at FES of 4 for 80 minutes.
- **Run #4:** Continue the run at FES of 4 for 35 minutes and finish with 45 minutes at FES of 5.

FIRST Exertion Scale (FES)

1	Very easy and relaxed
2	Relaxed effort with a slight increase in heart rate
3	A steady aerobic effort with breathing normal
4	Aware of effort but not experiencing any difficulties
5	Not laboring but having to stay focused to maintain effort
6	Having to coax yourself to maintain intensity
7	Comfortably hard; audible breathing; conversation has ceased
8	Heavy breathing; really hard effort
9	Very heavy breathing; can sustain only for a few minutes
10	Very, very hard; maximal effort

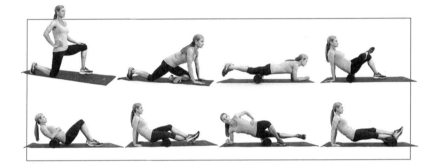

STRETCHES (AFTER RUN, 15 MINUTES)

(For images and information on these stretches, see Chapter 13.)

Open High Kneel
- 45 seconds each leg

Pigeon Pose
- 45 seconds each leg

Quadriceps with Roller
- 60 seconds

Piriformis Stretch with Roller
- 60 seconds each side

Lower Back with Roller
- 60 seconds

Hamstrings with Roller
- 60 seconds each side

ITB with Roller
- 60 seconds each side

Gastrocnemius with Roller
- 60 seconds each side

SUNDAY:
Cross-Train 30 Minutes, Stretch 10 Minutes

CROSS-TRAINING WORKOUTS (CHOOSE ONE)

Cycling Workout #1
- Begin with 10 minutes of cycling at cadence of 80+ rpm at FES of 2.
- 8 x (1 minute hard at FES of 7, 1 minute easy at FES of 2).
- 4 minutes of cycling at FES of 2 as a cooldown.

Cycling Workout #2
- Begin with 5 minutes of cycling at cadence of 80+ rpm at FES of 2.
- 4 x (1 minute fast at FES of 7, 1 minute at FES of 2).
- 1 x (4 minutes fast at FES of 7, 1 minute at FES of 2).
- 4 x (1 minute fast at FES of 7, 1 minute at FES of 2).
- 4 minutes of cycling at FES of 2 as a cooldown.

Rowing Workout
- 5 minutes of rowing at FES of 3 as a warmup.
- 6 x (500 meters at FES of 7, 1 minute at FES of 2).
- 2 minutes of easy rowing at FES of 2 as a cooldown.

Elliptical Workout
- 4 minutes at FES of 3 as a warmup.
- 8 x (2 minutes fast at FES of 7, 1-minute recovery at FES of 2).
- 2 minutes at FES of 2 as a cooldown.

FIRST Exertion Scale (FES)

1	Very easy and relaxed
2	Relaxed effort with a slight increase in heart rate
3	A steady aerobic effort with breathing normal
4	Aware of effort but not experiencing any difficulties
5	Not laboring but having to stay focused to maintain effort
6	Having to coax yourself to maintain intensity
7	Comfortably hard; audible breathing; conversation has ceased
8	Heavy breathing; really hard effort
9	Very heavy breathing; can sustain only for a few minutes
10	Very, very hard; maximal effort

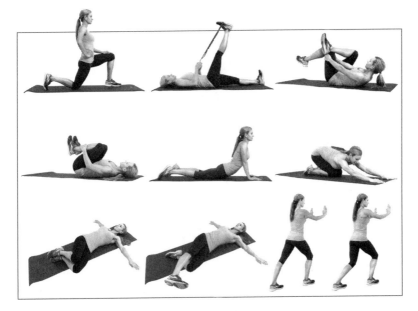

STRETCHES (10 MINUTES)

(For images and information on these stretches, see Chapter 13.)

Tall Kneeling Stretch
- 30 seconds each side

Hamstring with Rope
- 30 seconds each side

Piriformis Stretch
- 30 seconds each side

Lower-Back Stretch #1
- 30 seconds

Cobra/Prone Back Extension
- 30 seconds

Lower-Back Stretch #2
- 30 seconds

Spinal Rotation
- 30 seconds each side

Hip Abductors/ITB with Spinal Rotation
- 30 seconds each side

Isolated Gastrocnemius Stretch
- 30 seconds each leg

Isolated Soleus Stretch
- 30 seconds each leg

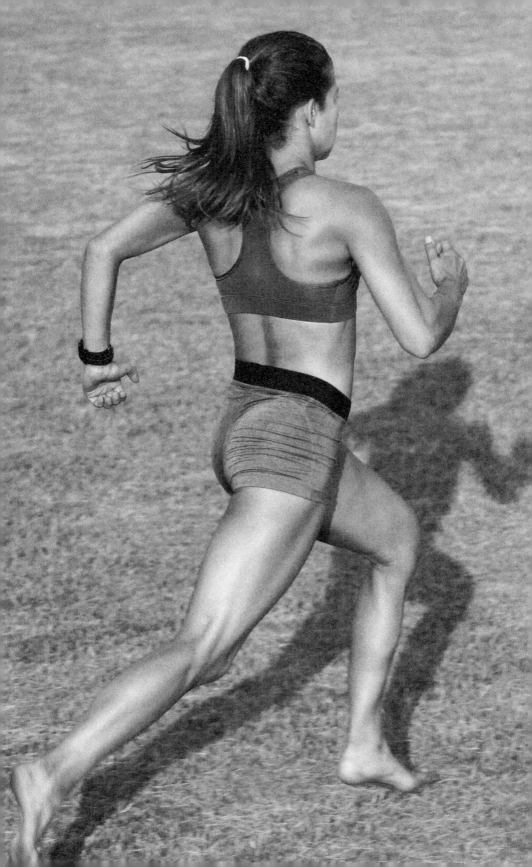

CHAPTER **12**

STRENGTH TRAINING: ESSENTIAL FOR LIFELONG RUNNING

IF YOU WISH TO BE healthy, fit, and fast, you must include strength training in your regular exercise routine. We are aware that many runners do not—as evidenced by their poor posture and inability to do resistance exercises. Maintaining muscle mass is important for reducing injury risk, for enhancing physical performance, for maintaining or improving body composition, and for maintaining overall good health. Without strengthening exercises, muscle mass shrinks with age; balance, agility, and coordination diminish as a result.

A strong musculature can better absorb the stressful impact of repetitive footstrikes on the body. Without adequate muscle mass for the absorption, bones and connective tissue suffer. Stress fractures are much more common among thin runners. The more the muscles absorb the shock, the less the bones need to do so.

Strengthening the calf will reduce stress on the ankle and tibia, while strengthening the quadriceps and hamstrings will reduce stress on the femur.

Running speed is determined by stride length and stride frequency. Stride length increases if there is more strength available in the push-off phase of the gait. Having more strength comes from being stronger from the hips and lower extremities. Resistance training develops muscle strength, which provides more strength during the push-off phase of the running cycle.

As we age, we lose type II, or fast-twitch, muscle fibers more quickly than we lose slow-twitch fibers. Strength training helps retain fast-twitch fibers, which can contribute to a runner's ability to run fast.[1] We all want to be able to sprint to the finish line.

Too many runners are worried about total body weight, when in fact they need to be more concerned about their body composition.

Strength, or resistance, training contributes to producing more lean mass. In particular, runners begin to lose muscle mass sometime in their thirties. Runners can raise their fitness level by increasing their musculature.

The American College of Sports Medicine recommends that adults perform resistance exercises for each of the major muscle group two or more times per week. Without the strength to perform daily tasks, independent living may not be possible. Studies show that performing resistance exercises can increase muscle mass even for people in their eighties and nineties.[2]

The strength-training exercises included in the 7-Hour Workout Week are described beginning on page 173. The order of the particular exercises and suggested number of repetitions or duration are indicated in the 7-Hour Workout Week plan.

Strength-Training Exercises

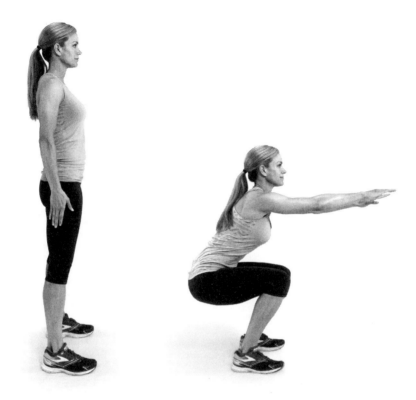

BODY-WEIGHT SQUAT

- Stand with your feet shoulder width apart and your arms down by your sides.
- Keeping your back straight, core tight, and knees pointing in the same direction as your feet, squat down, bending at your hips and knees until your thighs are parallel to the floor.
- Keep your weight on your heels rather than on the front of your foot so your knees do not extend beyond your toes.
- Place your hands on your hips or extend your arms out in front to help maintain your balance.
- In a controlled movement, return to the starting position by extending the knees and hips until you are standing in an upright position.

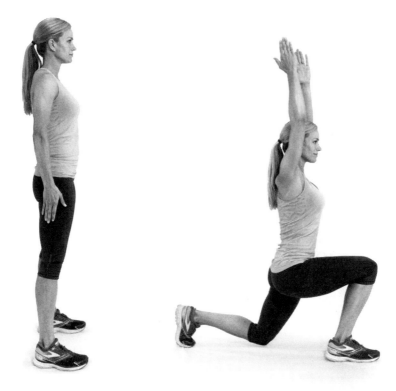

WALKING LUNGES WITH HANDS OVERHEAD

- Begin standing with your feet shoulder width apart and your arms by your sides.
- Maintaining an upright posture, raise your arms overhead and take a step forward with your right leg, landing on your right heel as you bend your knees in a forward lunge.
- Your front thigh should be parallel to the floor. Keep your back knee from touching the ground.
- Avoid stepping so far forward that your front knee extends beyond the point of your front toes. Your lead knee should point in the same direction as your foot throughout the lunge.
- Push off with your forward foot to bring your back leg forward, stepping into a lunge on your left side.
- Continue stepping forward, alternating legs the prescribed number of reps for each leg.

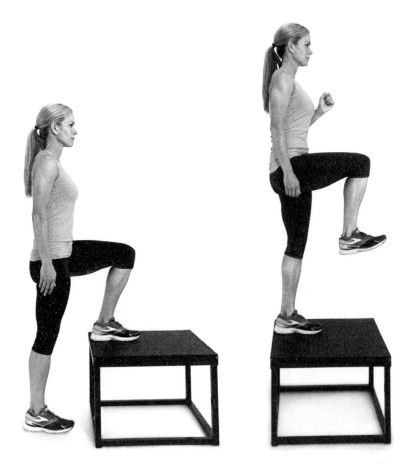

BOX STEPUPS

- Find a box with a height so that when your foot is on top of the box, your thigh is parallel to the ground.
- Use your left leg to raise yourself up by extending your left hip and knee to stand up on top of the box.
- Use your left leg to lift the rest of your body up and try to avoid pushing up with your right foot.
- Step down with the right leg and return to the original standing position. Repeat with the left leg for the prescribed repetitions, then switch to the right leg for the required repetitions.
- Keep your torso upright during the box stepups. Your forward knee should point in the same direction as your foot.

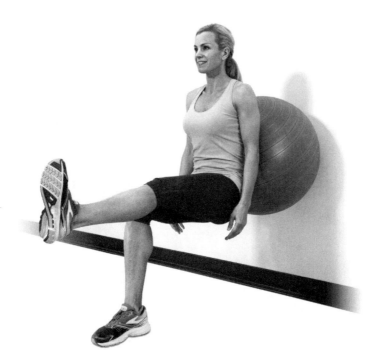

SINGLE-LEG WALL SQUAT WITH EXERCISE BALL

- Stand with your feet shoulder width apart and place an exercise ball against the wall at mid-back height. Stabilize the ball between your back and the wall.

- Take a step out from the wall so you can bend your knees to a 90-degree angle, keeping your knees over your ankles.

- Straighten your right knee. Lift your left leg off the floor as you bend your right knee to 90 degrees with your left leg off the floor.

- Your supporting knee should point in the same direction as your supporting foot.

- The ball will roll up your back as you squat down with your knee. Try to make sure that you do not arch your back. Your knee should not extend beyond the end of your toes.

- Repeat the exercise, squatting on the left leg with the right leg lifted off the floor.

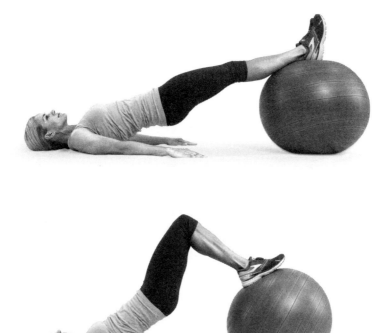

HIP EXTENSION LEG CURL WITH EXERCISE BALL

- Lie on your back on the floor with your feet on top of an exercise ball and your arms by your sides.
- Position the ball so that when your legs are straight, your ankles are on top of the ball.
- Raise your hips off the ground, keeping your weight on your shoulder blades and your feet until your body forms a straight line from shoulders to heels. This is your starting position.
- Keep your hips high and pull your heels and the exercise ball toward your butt until your feet are flat on the ball.
- Keep your glutes tight and avoid dropping your butt toward the ground.
- Keeping your hips high, let the ball roll back slowly as you straighten your legs and return to the starting position.

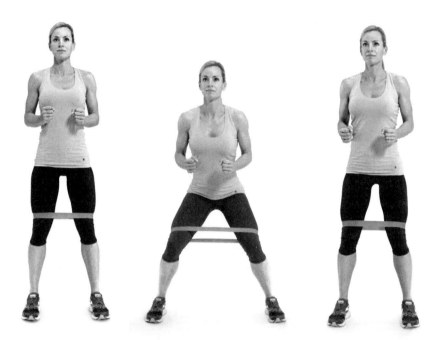

LATERAL STEPS WITH MINIBAND

- Place a miniband above your knees (you can lower the miniband toward your ankles as you improve your strength).
- Stand with your feet shoulder width apart to create tension on the band. Maintain an upright posture and look straight ahead. Your toes should be facing forward and your feet parallel.
- Stand with your knees slightly bent and step laterally with one foot and then bring the other leg inward to a new ready position, maintaining tension of the resistance band.
- Step to the right for the prescribed number of repetitions, then step to the left for the prescribed number of steps.
- Always keep tension on the band when you are stepping, and do not let your feet come together. Keep your feet pointed straight forward during the entire exercise.

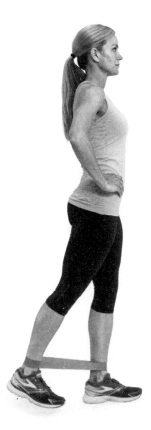

KICKBACKS WITH MINIBAND

- Place a miniband just above your ankles.
- Face a wall or use a chair to keep upright and maintain your balance.
- Slightly bend your left leg while you lift the right foot just off the ground. Keep your right leg straight and drive your right foot back behind you.
- Keep your body upright throughout the movement and avoid leaning forward in order to get the leg farther up behind you.
- With a controlled motion, pause at the back of the leg swing and then return to the starting position. Repeat on the same side for the prescribed number of repetitions, then switch sides.

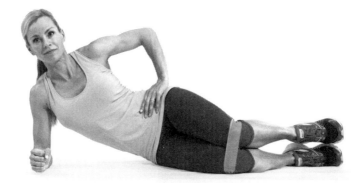

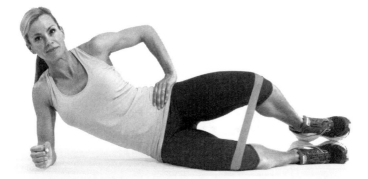

CLAMSHELL WITH MINIBAND

- Place a miniband around your legs just above your knees.
- Lie on your right side, propped up on your forearm, with your left leg stacked on top of your right leg and your knees bent at a 45-degree angle. Your heels should be in line with your butt.
- Raise your top knee toward the ceiling as high as you can. Keep your feet together and avoid rotating your pelvis or back. Your lower leg remains on the floor during the exercise.
- Hold for a second at the top, then slowly lower your knee to the starting position.

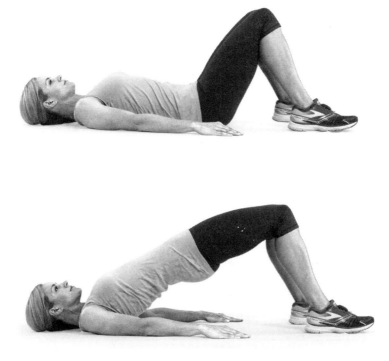

BRIDGE/PELVIC THRUST WITH FEET FLAT

- Lie on your back with your feet flat on the floor directly under your knees.
- Place your arms at your sides, with the palms on the floor next to your hips.
- Pressing into the floor with your hands and feet, exhale as you tighten the hamstring and gluteal muscles and lift your pelvis upward to form a straight line from shoulders to knees.
- Make sure you are driving straight up and your knees stay apart.
- Pause for 1 second, then slowly lower your hips toward the ground but not all the way.

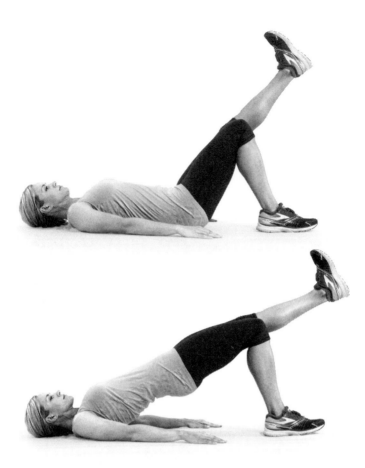

SINGLE-LEG BRIDGE/PELVIC THRUST

- Lie on your back with your feet flat on the floor directly under your knees.
- Place your arms at your sides, with the palms on the floor next to your hips.
- Straighten your left leg and hold it even with the right leg.
- Keeping the right foot flat on the ground, press into the floor with your hands and feet, exhale, and lift your pelvis upward to form a straight line from shoulders to knee.
- Make sure you are driving straight up and your knees stay apart.
- Pause for 1 second, then slowly lower the hips toward the ground but not all the way.
- Repeat the exercise with the opposite leg.

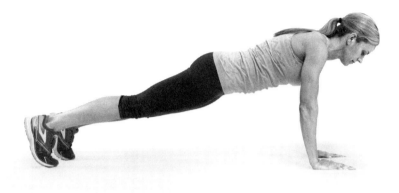

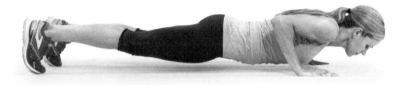

PUSHUPS (STANDARD OR MODIFIED)

- Get into a high plank position with your hands on the ground, directly under your shoulders. Brace your core (tighten your abs), keeping your back straight.
- Lower your body, keeping your back straight, until your chest grazes the floor. Do not let your hips sag or point up.
- Your body should remain in a straight line from head to toe.
- Keeping your body straight, exhale as you push back up to the starting position.
- Keep your hips straight throughout the entire movement.

MODIFIED: Perform the exercise with the knees on the floor, keeping your hips straight.

MORE ADVANCED: Perform the pushups on a BOSU ball.

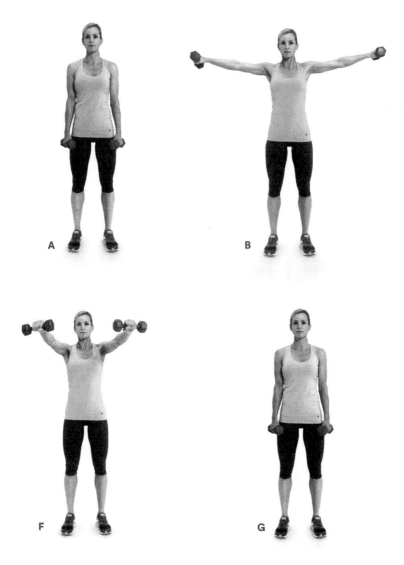

A

B

F

G

DUMBBELL CLOCKER SHOULDER RAISE

- Visualize the body as the center of a clock and you are facing 12 o'clock.
- Stand holding a pair of dumbbells by your side and raise your arms to the 3 o'clock and 9 o'clock positions until your arms are just slightly above horizontal. Then lower.
- Raise your arms to the 2 o'clock and 10 o'clock positions, then lower.

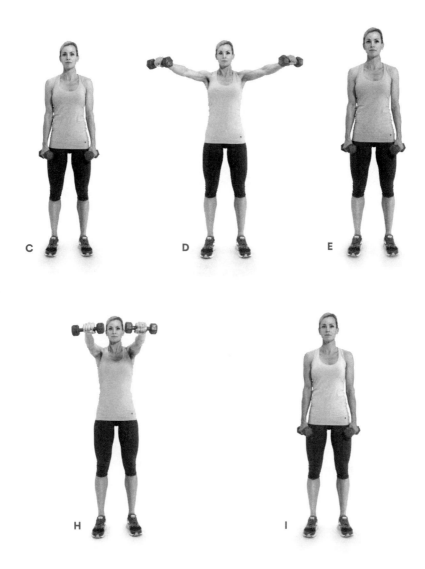

- Raise your arms to the 1 o'clock and 11 o'clock positions, then lower.
- Raise your arms to the 12 o'clock position, then lower.
- Repeat this sequence 4 more times.

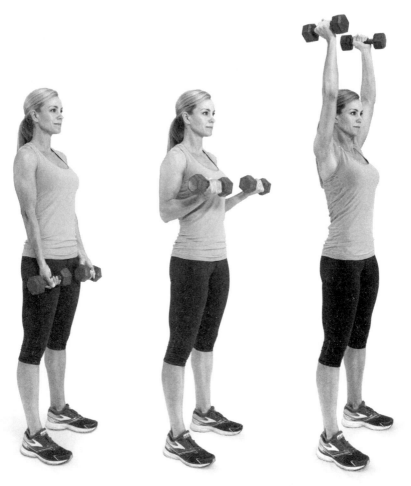

DUMBBELL CURL TO PRESS

- Stand straight, holding a dumbbell in each hand with your arms extended down and by your sides. Keeping your upper arms and elbows stationary and close to your torso with your palms facing forward, curl the dumbbells up toward your shoulders.
- Press the weights over your head, rotating as you go so your palms face each other at the top of the movement.
- Avoid arching your back as you press the weight overhead.
- Lower both arms with control and return the arms to the curl position, then lower to the starting position.

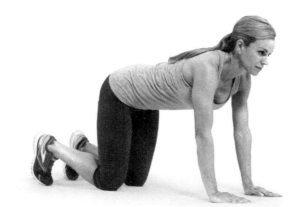

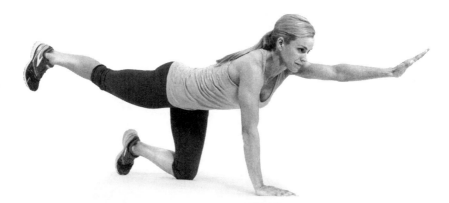

QUADRUPED/POINTER DOG

- On a mat, start on all fours with your hands under your shoulders and your knees under your hips. Your head, neck, and back should be straight.
- During the exercise, keep your head level, not raised upward, in a neutral position to minimize pressure on your neck.
- Raise your left arm and reach forward until it is in line with your torso.
- As you bring your left arm forward, straighten and lift your right leg up until it is straight and in line with your torso. Hold this position for 3 seconds.
- Slowly bring your left arm and right leg back to the ground and repeat with the right arm and left leg.

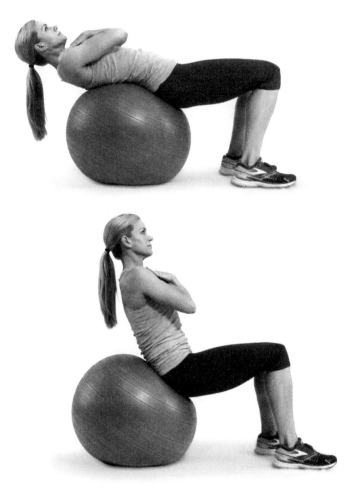

ABDOMINAL CRUNCH ON EXERCISE BALL

- Sit on an exercise ball and place your feet flat on the floor, shoulder width apart. Roll back until your lower back is resting comfortably on the ball. Position your arms across your chest with your hands near your shoulders. Raise your head even with your torso, looking straight up.

- Contract your abs and slowly curl your torso forward to raise your chest up and to an upright or vertical position. Raise your chest until you feel your abs completely contract; pause for 1 second and lower your head and torso back to the starting position.

- Perform the crunches in a controlled manner and avoid bouncing on the ball; focus on your abs while doing the exercise.

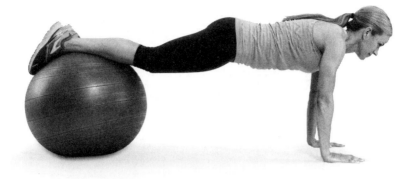

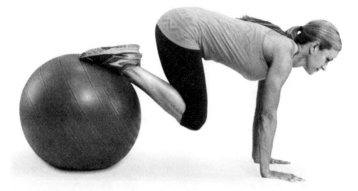

REVERSE CRUNCH WITH EXERCISE BALL

- Lie on an exercise ball on your stomach, with your feet touching the floor behind the ball.
- Lean forward until you touch the floor with your hands.
- Walk your hands away from the ball until you feel the ball reach your lower legs.
- Keep your shoulders directly above your hands. Keeping your hands in place, use your abdominal muscles to roll the ball forward by bending your knees and hips.
- Hold this position for a second and roll back out.

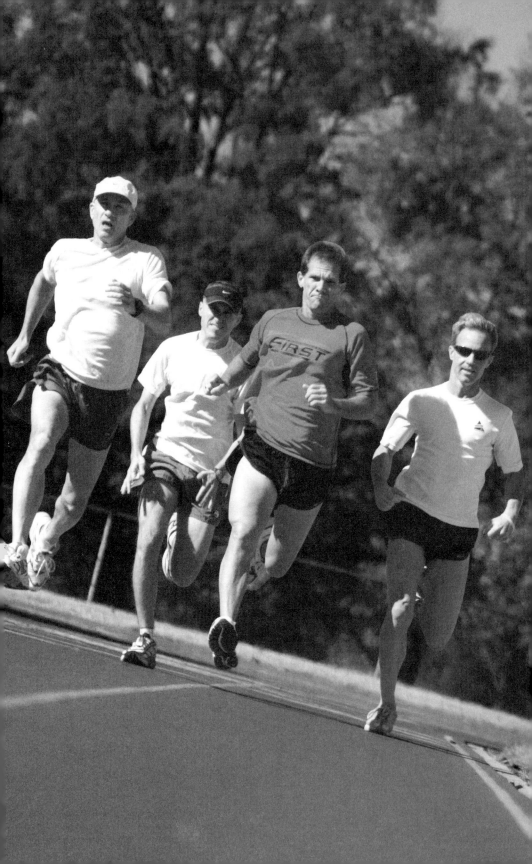

CHAPTER 13

STRETCHING: ESSENTIAL FOR LIFELONG RUNNING

TO STRETCH OR NOT TO stretch? That is a common question among runners and researchers. Studies yield conflicting answers regarding the effects of stretching on performance and the value of stretching for injury prevention. At FIRST, we believe that stretching is an important component of fitness training.

Flexibility is determined by the range of motion across a joint or multiple joints. It is influenced by age, gender, genetics, injuries, activity level, temperature, and time of day. Joint range of motion and muscle flexibility are foundations of functional performance. The American College of Sports Medicine (ACSM) includes flexibility as a component of fitness.

The risk factors associated with poor flexibility include faulty posture, altered running mechanics, impaired running economy, and risk of injury and pain. At our FIRST retreats, we commonly see poor posture among runners with poor flexibility. That poor posture contributes to poor running form, which in turn contributes to inefficiency and, yes, slower times.

Poor posture or form causes a runner to expend more energy to maintain a given pace. That causes the runner to be less economical. Using more oxygen and glycogen because of poor mechanics means that the runner is not fulfilling his potential.

A common problem among runners is restricted ankle flexibility. This lack of ankle range of motion, especially the inability to pull toes toward the shin, results in lower-extremity injuries—calves, knees, hamstrings, hips—by transferring stress and impact to these lower-extremity sites. Stretching to improve ankle flexibility should be a part of every runner's workout routine.

Because runners typically lose flexibility as they age, a common characteristic of the older runner is a stride that becomes shorter than optimal. However, shortened strides are not limited to older runners. Any runner with tight hamstrings and a tight lower back will have a shortened stride, which impairs running economy.

The potential benefits from stretching include:

❱ Increased range of motion

❱ Reduced risk of injury

❱ Enhanced performance

❱ Improved body alignment

❱ Reduced muscular tension

Conflicting Interpretation of Studies of Stretching

If there are significant benefits from stretching, including an increased range of motion, why is there controversy and conflicting evidence about the merits of stretching? Here are what we at FIRST see as the reasons for the confusion. First, a common research design is to divide runners into two groups—one is assigned to a training group that stretches and the other to a training group that does not stretch. Otherwise, their running training is identical. The runners are tested by having them run a time trial before and after a training period typically of 12 to 16 weeks. If there are no statistically significant differences in performance improvements of the two groups, it is concluded that stretching did not improve running performance.

The flaw in such studies that compare runners who stretch with runners who do not is that stretching and improved joint mobility do not immediately affect running performance, particularly in distance running. Without longitudinal studies measuring runners' flexibility over years, we are not likely to see the real impact of a steadfast commitment to stretching.

The other factor fueling the stretching controversy comes from studies that survey runners to ask if they stretch. The survey results are analyzed to see if runners who stretch are more likely to be injured than those who do not stretch. The problem with this research approach is that runners who are injured are likely to begin stretching to address their injuries, either on their own or as directed by a physical therapist. In other words, the stretching is done to treat an injury, not to prevent one.

How to Use Stretching to Improve Fitness

FIRST is strongly committed to stretching. Three types of stretching can be utilized by runners to reduce injuries and improve performance: static stretching, dynamic stretching, and proprioceptive neuromuscular facilitation (PNF) stretching. Static stretching is performed by holding a stretch without movement. Dynamic stretching is performed by gentle swinging motion to the limits of nonpainful stretching. PNF stretching is a series of muscular contractions followed by relaxation to gradually increase the range of motion.

The best fitness routines include all three types of stretching. Dynamic stretching is recommended as a preperformance warmup. Static stretching should be performed after running, later in the day, or on nonrunning days. PNF stretching, which is often performed with a partner or trainer, is typically performed after working out.

Professional athletes commonly have a trainer who stretches them after each workout. Runners who run with a partner can assist each other with stretching. Another method of ensuring regular stretching is to attend a yoga class.

The foam roller is an alternative method for stretching through self-massage, referred to as self-myofascial release. It enables the runner to relieve tightness and stiffness. Newer rollers are much firmer than the original models. Some have grooves and even thumblike projections to provide massagelike pressure. With a little practice, you can move the roller into positions to massage the entire body and thus place pressure on trigger points and relieve muscular tightness. Other stretching accessories, such as massage sticks and therapy balls, can provide similar relief.

The goal of any runner is to develop symmetrical strength and flexibility, stable running form, and pain-free, injury-free running. A consistent habit of stretching should be included in a runner's workout routine. The ACSM recommends completing a series of flexibility exercises for each major muscle-tendon group two or more times per week.

We have included daily stretching, detailed in the following pages, in the 7-Hour Workout Week. Do not skip it.

On days when you run, we suggest 5 minutes of dynamic stretching (five dynamic stretches) before your run and 10 to 15 minutes of stretching after your run (eight stretches).

On the nonrunning days, we suggest 10 minutes of stretching after your workout (six to nine different stretches).

Stretching Exercises
Dynamic Stretches Before Your Run (about 5 minutes)

Focus on a controlled motion while working toward increasing your available range of motion.

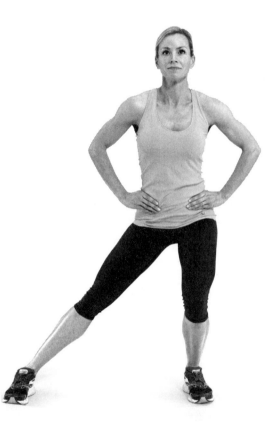

DYNAMIC SIDE LUNGE

- Keeping the feet facing forward, take a wide step out to your left side.
- Let your left hip and knee bend with your body weight over your left foot.
- Keep your right leg straight. Push back up to the starting position and alternate to the other side and repeat.

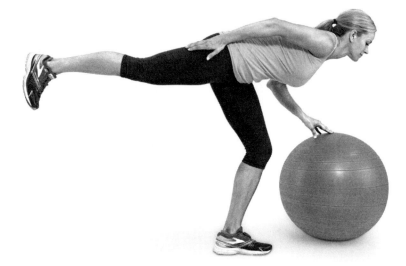

DYNAMIC SINGLE-LEG DEADLIFT

- Stand on your left leg with a slight bend in your knee.
- Keeping your spine straight and your right leg straight and in line with your torso, slowly bend forward at the hip and lower your upper body until your torso and right leg are parallel to the floor.
- Return to the upright position and repeat for 30 seconds, then switch to your right leg and repeat for 30 seconds.

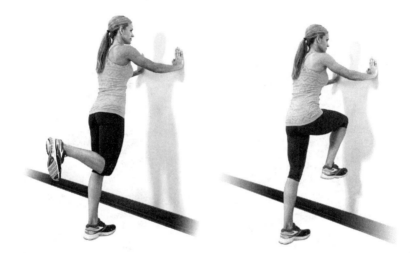

DYNAMIC BENT-KNEE FORWARD SWING

- Facing a wall, lean slightly forward at your waist and place your hands on the wall for support.
- With one knee bent at a 90-degree angle, drive this knee up toward your chest to a comfortable height in a rhythmical and controlled motion.
- Gradually increase the range of motion until the leg swings as high as it will comfortably go.
- Repeat with the other leg.

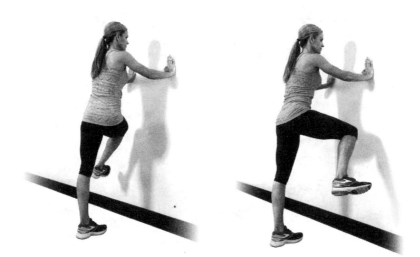

DYNAMIC BENT-KNEE LATERAL SWING

- Facing a wall, lean slightly forward at your waist and place your hands on the wall for support.
- With one knee bent at a 90-degree angle, drive this knee up and across your torso toward the opposite shoulder and then up and out toward the other shoulder.
- Gradually increase the range of motion until the leg swings as high as it will comfortably go.
- Repeat with the other leg.

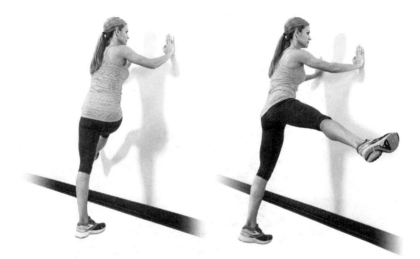

DYNAMIC STRAIGHT-LEG LATERAL SWING

- Facing a wall, lean slightly forward at your waist and place your hands on the wall for support.
- Keeping your knee straight and leading with the heel, alternate swinging your leg out and away from the body and then across the front of the body in a rhythmical motion.
- Gradually increase the range of motion until the leg swings as high as it will comfortably go.
- Repeat with the other leg.

Stretches After Your Run (10–15 minutes)

Try to stretch beyond your available range of motion but not to the point of pain. Hold each stretch for 30–45 seconds.

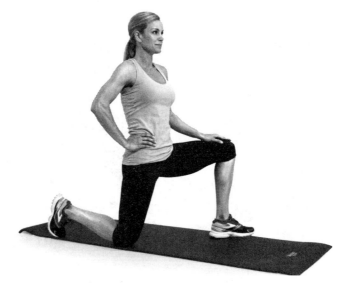

RUN TRAINING DAY STRETCH #1

OPEN HIGH KNEEL

- Kneel on the ground on your right knee and place your left foot in front of your body.
- Rotate your left leg 90 degrees out to your left side.
- Press your hips forward, keeping your torso straight and your core tight.
- Hold the stretch for 30–45 seconds, then switch sides.

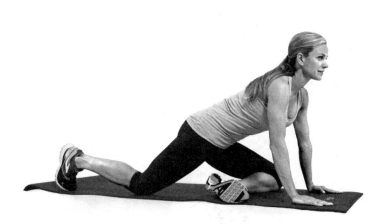

PIGEON POSE

- Place your right leg straight behind you and your left leg crossed in front of your body.
- Your left shin may angle back toward the right hip or be more parallel to the front of your mat, depending on your flexibility.
- Keep the front of your left leg as flat on the floor as possible.
- Keep your hips square and facing the front of your mat.
- Support your torso with your hands on the ground in front of you.
- Lean your torso forward, keeping your core tight.
- Hold the stretch for 30–45 seconds, then switch sides.

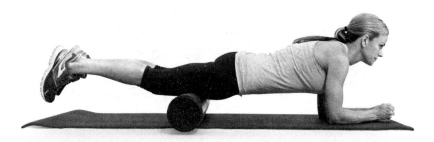

RUN TRAINING DAY STRETCH #3

QUADRICEPS WITH ROLLER

- Lie facedown with a foam roller positioned near your hips while supporting yourself on your elbows.
- Keep your core tight and your torso straight.
- Using your arms, slowly move your body forward and backward, allowing the foam roller to roll slowly across your thighs.
- You can either do both legs at the same time or one leg at a time. By doing one leg at a time, you can target different angles on the foam roller by turning your feet both in and out.
- Gently roll back and forth for 30–45 seconds.

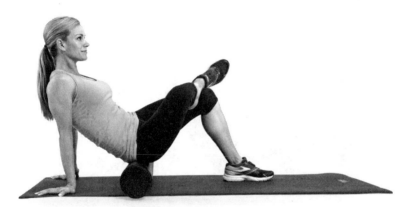

RUN TRAINING DAY STRETCH #4

PIRIFORMIS STRETCH WITH ROLLER

- Sit on a foam roller and place your right ankle on your left knee.
- Lean back slightly with your body weight over your right hip.
- Slowly roll back and forth over the right hip, using your arms and supporting leg to control the pressure to focus on any tender areas.
- Gently roll back and forth for 30–45 seconds, then switch sides.

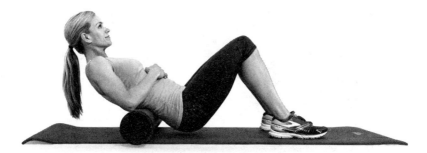

RUN TRAINING DAY STRETCH #5

LOWER BACK WITH ROLLER

- Lie on the floor with your arms in front of your chest and a foam roller positioned against your lower back.
- Lift your hips up off the ground, then slowly roll across your lower back.
- Turn slightly to the left and right if there is too much pressure on your spine.
- Gently roll back and forth for 30–45 seconds.

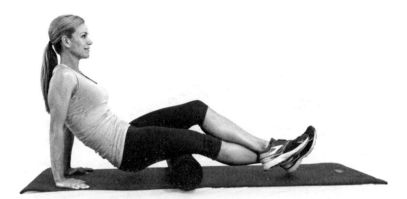

RUN TRAINING DAY STRETCH #6

HAMSTRINGS WITH ROLLER

- Position a foam roller under your thighs while using your arms to help hold your hips off the ground.
- Roll back and forth slowly across your hamstrings, focusing on any tender areas.
- Roll with your feet turned in and out to cover the entire muscle group.
- For a more advanced stretch, stack your legs to increase the weight on the bottom leg, then switch sides.
- Gently roll back and forth for 30–45 seconds.

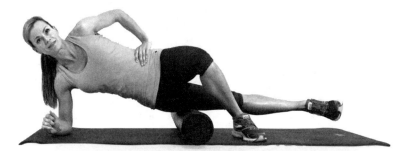

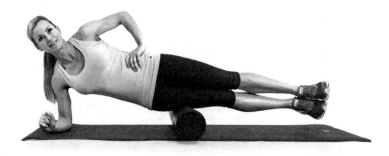

RUN TRAINING DAY STRETCH #7

ITB WITH ROLLER

- Lie on your side using your forearm to support your upper body.
- Place a foam roller under your mid-thigh with the foot of the lower leg off the ground.
- Roll slowly along the length of your thigh.
- Keep your opposite foot on the ground for support.
- For a more advanced stretch, stack both legs so there is more weight on the roller.
- Gently roll back and forth for 30–45 seconds, then switch sides.

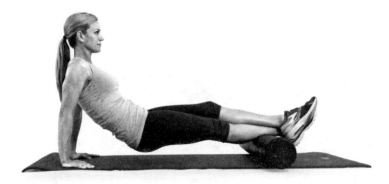

RUN TRAINING DAY STRETCH #8

GASTROCNEMIUS WITH ROLLER

- Position a foam roller under one calf while using your arms to support your weight.
- Roll back and forth slowly across the calf.
- Roll from your ankle to just below your knee to target the entire muscle.
- Gently roll back and forth for 30–45 seconds, then switch sides.
- Focus extra time on tender areas.

Try to stretch beyond your available range of motion but not to the point of pain. Hold stretches for 30–45 seconds.

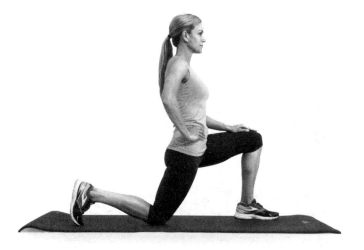

CROSS-TRAINING DAY STRETCH #1

TALL KNEELING STRETCH

- Kneel on the ground on your right knee, and place your left foot in front of your body.
- Press your hips forward, keeping your torso straight and your core tight.
- Your forward knee should not extend beyond the point of your toes.
- Hold the stretch for 30–45 seconds, then switch sides.

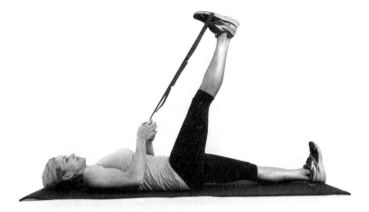

CROSS-TRAINING DAY STRETCH #2

HAMSTRING WITH ROPE

- Lie on the floor on your back with your legs straight forward.
- Using a rope or strap around the arch of your right foot, lift your right leg as far as you can toward the ceiling, keeping your knee and leg straight. Use the rope for gentle assistance at the end of the stretch.
- Lower the leg and repeat, trying to lift your leg a little higher.
- For a more advanced hamstring stretch, tighten the hamstrings of the elevated leg to push down into the rope. Resist with your arms while maintaining a static position. Tighten your hamstrings for 10 seconds, then relax and attempt to pull the elevated leg further toward your torso for an additional stretch.
- Hold the stretch for 30–45 seconds, then switch sides.

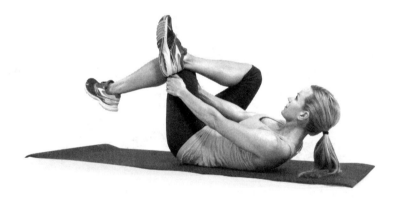

CROSS-TRAINING DAY STRETCH #3

PIRIFORMIS STRETCH

- Lie on the floor on your back with your knees bent and your feet flat on the floor.
- Bend your right leg and place the ankle in front of your left knee.
- Clasp both hands behind your left thigh and pull your legs toward your torso until a stretch is felt in the right hip and glutes.
- Hold the stretch for 30–45 seconds, then switch sides.

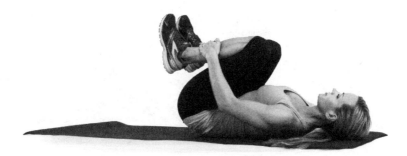

CROSS-TRAINING DAY STRETCH #4

LOWER-BACK STRETCH #1

- Lie on the floor on your back with your knees bent and your feet flat on the floor.
- Slowly bring your knees toward your chest and gently grasp your legs below the knee.
- Hold them in place for 30–45 seconds and avoid rocking back and forth.

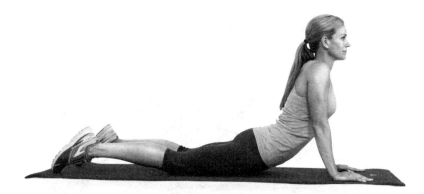

CROSS-TRAINING DAY STRETCH #5

COBRA/PRONE BACK EXTENSION

- Begin in a facedown position on the floor with your palms flat, placed beneath your shoulders.

- Tighten your abs and draw your belly button toward your spine. You want to engage your abs to protect your lower back.

- Spread your fingers and press your palms into the floor.

- Push your upper body off the floor and straighten your arms as much as is comfortable while keeping your hips, legs, and feet stationary on the floor. Your lower back will be slightly arched.

- Go only as far as comfortable, and stop if you experience any pain. Hold the stretch for 30–45 seconds.

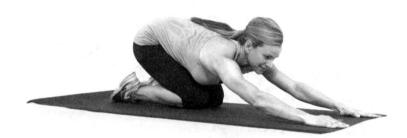

CROSS-TRAINING DAY STRETCH #6

LOWER-BACK STRETCH #2

- On your hands and knees, drop your hips back until your glutes rest on your heels.
- Lower your chest to the floor and stretch your arms out straight in front of you. Hold the stretch for 30-45 seconds.

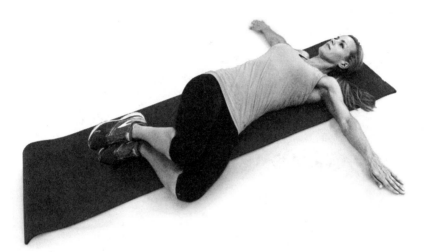

CROSS-TRAINING DAY STRETCH #7

SPINAL ROTATION

- Lie on the floor on your back. Bend your knees and keep your feet flat on the floor.
- Extend your arms at shoulder level.
- Slowly let your knees fall toward your left side until a gentle stretch is felt in your back.
- Keep your knees together during the stretch.
- Hold the stretch for 30–45 seconds, then switch sides.

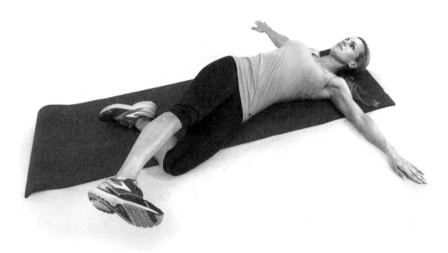

CROSS-TRAINING DAY STRETCH #8

HIP ABDUCTORS/ITB WITH SPINAL ROTATION

- Lie on the floor on your back. Bend your knees and keep your feet flat on the floor.
- Extend your arms at shoulder level.
- Slowly let your knees fall toward your left side until a gentle stretch is felt in your back.
- Keep your knees together during the stretch.
- Extend the top leg out straight (you can use a rope or strap to gently pull your straight leg so that it becomes perpendicular to your torso). Hold the stretch for 30–45 seconds, then switch sides.

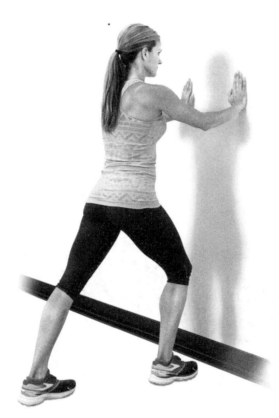

CROSS-TRAINING DAY STRETCH #9

ISOLATED GASTROCNEMIUS STRETCH

- Facing a wall, place your left leg back behind you with the toes of your back foot slightly toed in.
- Bend your front leg to lean forward against the wall.
- Press your hips toward the wall while keeping your back leg straight and your heel flat on the ground. Hold the stretch for 30–45 seconds, then switch legs.

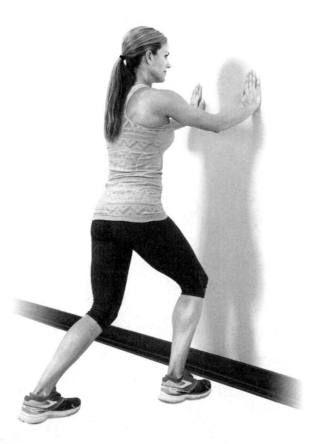

CROSS-TRAINING DAY STRETCH #10

ISOLATED SOLEUS STRETCH

- Facing a wall, place your left leg back behind you with the toes of your back foot slightly toed in.
- Bend your front leg to lean forward against the wall.
- After performing the gastrocnemius stretch, press your hips toward the wall and stretch the soleus by slightly bending the knee of your back leg.
- Maintain this position as you press your hips toward the wall while keeping your heel flat on the ground. Hold the stretch for 30–45 seconds, then switch legs.

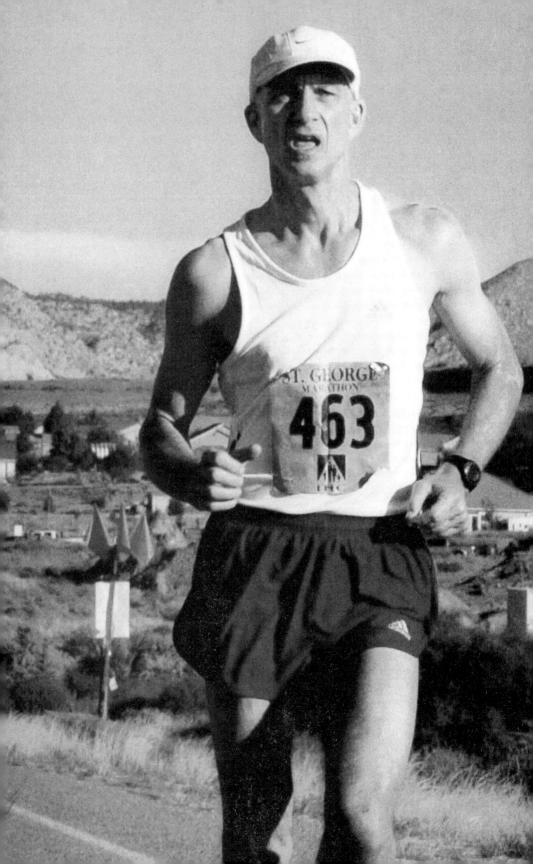

AFTERWORD

SCOTT, DON, AND I TRAIN using the 7-Hour Workout Week. We are just as susceptible to the loss of core strength and flexibility as any other aging runner. The program is not short on intensity, and we have used it to prepare for marathons, half-marathons, and 5-K races.

What is it like to follow the 7-Hour Workout Week? I find it refreshing. I definitely need a structured strengthening and stretching program. While I did a variety of exercises in the past, they were not carefully chosen. I have become committed to the small number of specific strength exercises and stretches specified in the workout. I am less likely to skip this important nonrunning aspect of my overall training when it is specifically prescribed and time manageable.

What is it like to perform the run workouts using perceived exertion? I still wear a watch but not to time-fixed intervals. When I go out to run fast repeats on Tuesdays, I use the watch to let me know when the interval of 2, 3, 4, or 5 minutes of hard running is complete. The watch also tells me when my recovery interval is over. My intensity during those short 2- to 5-minute intervals is determined by my perceived exertion. I know those are to be done at a near all-out effort, so I focus on my form and breathing.

The tempo and long runs are intense efforts based on how many minutes I will be running. You gain a real sense of how hard you can run for 30 minutes, 60 minutes, or even 90 minutes. It also means that you do not have to run the same measured course, because you are running for total time. The workouts are no easier than running a specific distance with a specific goal time.

One, or all, of us generally wears a GPS watch on our long runs to record the distance and time. We do not use the information during the run to tell us to speed up or slow down. Rather than checking every mile split, we base our pace on effort and feel. Then one of us downloads the information after returning home, and we are able to see how our perceived effort compares to the paces we were maintaining during different phases of the workout.

This approach to training gives us the structure that we like and had become accustomed to when we were younger. Just like other runners, we still want to know what we are going to do after we have pulled on our running shoes.

The 7-Hour Workout Week works for us. Whether you use the time and perceived exertion training system for a few months in between race preparation training programs or whether you adopt it as your standard training program, we believe it will work for you.

APPENDIX A

PACE FOR RUN WORKOUTS

IF YOU PREFER PACE TO PERCEIVED EFFORT for the runs in Chapter 11, you can use these tables to find your needed run pace. You can use the times to set your Garmin or other training device. It's a simple two-step process. Use the minutes-per-kilometer table or the minutes-per-mile table, depending on how you prefer to think of your pace.

First, find the row that has your current 5-K run time. Second, look across the row to find the cell under your planned workout to find the pace you need to run. For example, if you are a 24-minute 5-K runner and want to do the 5-minute Tuesday workout, you will need to run at a pace of 4:35 per kilometer for 5 minutes. Or, if you think in miles per minute, you would need to run at a pace of 7:22 per mile for 5 minutes.

Minutes per Mile

5K TIME	TUESDAY		
	2 MIN. @	3 MIN. @	5 MIN.@
16:00	04:29	04:40	04:48
16:10	04:32	04:43	04:51
16:20	04:35	04:46	04:54
16:30	04:38	04:50	04:58
16:40	04:42	04:53	05:01
16:50	04:45	04:56	05:04
17:00	04:48	04:59	05:07
17:10	04:51	05:02	05:11
17:20	04:54	05:06	05:14
17:30	04:58	05:09	05:17
17:40	05:01	05:12	05:20
17:50	05:04	05:15	05:23
18:00	05:07	05:19	05:27
18:10	05:11	05:22	05:30
18:20	05:14	05:25	05:33
18:30	05:17	05:28	05:36
18:40	05:20	05:31	05:39
18:50	05:23	05:35	05:43
19:00	05:27	05:38	05:46
19:10	05:30	05:41	05:49
19:20	05:33	05:44	05:52
19:30	05:36	05:48	05:56
19:40	05:39	05:51	05:59
19:50	05:43	05:54	06:02
20:00	05:46	05:57	06:05
20:10	05:49	06:00	06:08
20:20	05:52	06:04	06:12
20:30	05:56	06:07	06:15
20:40	05:59	06:10	06:18
20:50	06:02	06:13	06:21
21:00	06:05	06:17	06:25
21:10	06:08	06:20	06:28
21:20	06:12	06:23	06:31
21:30	06:15	06:26	06:34
21:40	06:18	06:29	06:37

	THURSDAY			SATURDAY	
5K TIME	FES 7 TEMPO	FES 6 TEMPO	FES 5 TEMPO	FES 5 LONG	FES 4 LONG
16:00	05:25	05:41	05:57	06:15	06:26
16:10	05:28	05:44	06:00	06:18	06:29
16:20	05:31	05:48	06:04	06:21	06:33
16:30	05:35	05:51	06:07	06:25	06:36
16:40	05:38	05:54	06:10	06:28	06:39
16:50	05:41	05:57	06:13	06:31	06:42
17:00	05:44	06:00	06:17	06:34	06:45
17:10	05:48	06:04	06:20	06:37	06:49
17:20	05:51	06:07	06:23	06:41	06:52
17:30	05:54	06:10	06:26	06:44	06:55
17:40	05:57	06:13	06:29	06:47	06:58
17:50	06:00	06:17	06:33	06:50	07:02
18:00	06:04	06:20	06:36	06:54	07:05
18:10	06:07	06:23	06:39	06:57	07:08
18:20	06:10	06:26	06:42	07:00	07:11
18:30	06:13	06:29	06:45	07:03	07:14
18:40	06:17	06:33	06:49	07:06	07:18
18:50	06:20	06:36	06:52	07:10	07:21
19:00	06:23	06:39	06:55	07:13	07:24
19:10	06:26	06:42	06:58	07:16	07:27
19:20	06:29	06:45	07:02	07:19	07:31
19:30	06:33	06:49	07:05	07:22	07:34
19:40	06:36	06:52	07:08	07:26	07:37
19:50	06:39	06:55	07:11	07:29	07:40
20:00	06:42	06:58	07:14	07:32	07:43
20:10	06:45	07:02	07:18	07:35	07:47
20:20	06:49	07:05	07:21	07:39	07:50
20:30	06:52	07:08	07:24	07:42	07:53
20:40	06:55	07:11	07:27	07:45	07:56
20:50	06:58	07:14	07:31	07:48	07:59
21:00	07:02	07:18	07:34	07:51	08:03
21:10	07:05	07:21	07:37	07:55	08:06
21:20	07:08	07:24	07:40	07:58	08:09
21:30	07:11	07:27	07:43	08:01	08:12
21:40	07:14	07:31	07:47	08:04	08:16

Minutes per Mile

5K TIME	TUESDAY		
	2 MIN. @	3 MIN. @	5 MIN.@
21:50	06:21	06:33	06:41
22:00	06:25	06:36	06:44
22:10	06:28	06:39	06:47
22:20	06:31	06:42	06:50
22:30	06:34	06:45	06:54
22:40	06:37	06:49	06:57
22:50	06:41	06:52	07:00
23:00	06:44	06:55	07:03
23:10	06:47	06:58	07:06
23:20	06:50	07:02	07:10
23:30	06:54	07:05	07:13
23:40	06:57	07:08	07:16
23:50	07:00	07:11	07:19
24:00	07:03	07:14	07:22
24:10	07:06	07:18	07:26
24:20	07:10	07:21	07:29
24:30	07:13	07:24	07:32
24:40	07:16	07:27	07:35
24:50	07:19	07:31	07:39
25:00	07:22	07:34	07:42
25:10	07:26	07:37	07:45
25:20	07:29	07:40	07:48
25:30	07:32	07:43	07:51
25:40	07:35	07:47	07:55
25:50	07:39	07:50	07:58
26:00	07:42	07:53	08:01
26:10	07:45	07:56	08:04
26:20	07:48	07:59	08:08
26:30	07:51	08:03	08:11
26:40	07:55	08:06	08:14
26:50	07:58	08:09	08:17
27:00	08:01	08:12	08:20
27:10	08:04	08:16	08:24
27:20	08:08	08:19	08:27
27:30	08:11	08:22	08:30
27:40	08:14	08:25	08:33
27:50	08:17	08:28	08:36

	THURSDAY			SATURDAY	
5K TIME	FES 7 TEMPO	FES 6 TEMPO	FES 5 TEMPO	FES 5 LONG	FES 4 LONG
21:50	07:18	07:34	07:50	08:08	08:19
22:00	07:21	07:37	07:53	08:11	08:22
22:10	07:24	07:40	07:56	08:14	08:25
22:20	07:27	07:43	07:59	08:17	08:28
22:30	07:31	07:47	08:03	08:20	08:32
22:40	07:34	07:50	08:06	08:24	08:35
22:50	07:37	07:53	08:09	08:27	08:38
23:00	07:40	07:56	08:12	08:30	08:41
23:10	07:43	07:59	08:16	08:33	08:45
23:20	07:47	08:03	08:19	08:36	08:48
23:30	07:50	08:06	08:22	08:40	08:51
23:40	07:53	08:09	08:25	08:43	08:54
23:50	07:56	08:12	08:28	08:46	08:57
24:00	07:59	08:16	08:32	08:49	09:01
24:10	08:03	08:19	08:35	08:53	09:04
24:20	08:06	08:22	08:38	08:56	09:07
24:30	08:09	08:25	08:41	08:59	09:10
24:40	08:12	08:28	08:45	09:02	09:13
24:50	08:16	08:32	08:48	09:05	09:17
25:00	08:19	08:35	08:51	09:09	09:20
25:10	08:22	08:38	08:54	09:12	09:23
25:20	08:25	08:41	08:57	09:15	09:26
25:30	08:28	08:45	09:01	09:18	09:30
25:40	08:32	08:48	09:04	09:22	09:33
25:50	08:35	08:51	09:07	09:25	09:36
26:00	08:38	08:54	09:10	09:28	09:39
26:10	08:41	08:57	09:13	09:31	09:42
26:20	08:45	09:01	09:17	09:34	09:46
26:30	08:48	09:04	09:20	09:38	09:49
26:40	08:51	09:07	09:23	09:41	09:52
26:50	08:54	09:10	09:26	09:44	09:55
27:00	08:57	09:13	09:30	09:47	09:59
27:10	09:01	09:17	09:33	09:51	10:02
27:20	09:04	09:20	09:36	09:54	10:05
27:30	09:07	09:23	09:39	09:57	10:08
27:40	09:10	09:26	09:42	10:00	10:11
27:50	09:13	09:30	09:46	10:03	10:15

Minutes per Mile

5K TIME	TUESDAY		
	2 MIN. @	3 MIN. @	5 MIN.@
28:00	08:20	08:32	08:40
28:10	08:24	08:35	08:43
28:20	08:27	08:38	08:46
28:30	08:30	08:41	08:49
28:40	08:33	08:45	08:53
28:50	08:36	08:48	08:56
29:00	08:40	08:51	08:59
29:10	08:43	08:54	09:02
29:20	08:46	08:57	09:05
29:30	08:49	09:01	09:09
29:40	08:53	09:04	09:12
29:50	08:56	09:07	09:15
30:00	08:59	09:10	09:18
30:10	09:02	09:13	09:22
30:20	09:05	09:17	09:25
30:30	09:09	09:20	09:28
30:40	09:12	09:23	09:31
30:50	09:15	09:26	09:34
31:00	09:18	09:30	09:38
31:10	09:22	09:33	09:41
31:20	09:25	09:36	09:44
31:30	09:28	09:39	09:47
31:40	09:31	09:42	09:51
31:50	09:34	09:46	09:54
32:00	09:38	09:49	09:57
32:10	09:41	09:52	10:00
32:20	09:44	09:55	10:03
32:30	09:47	09:59	10:07
32:40	09:51	10:02	10:10
32:50	09:54	10:05	10:13
33:00	09:57	10:08	10:16
33:10	10:00	10:11	10:19
33:20	10:03	10:15	10:23
33:30	10:07	10:18	10:26
33:40	10:10	10:21	10:29
33:50	10:13	10:24	10:32
34:00	10:16	10:28	10:36

	THURSDAY			SATURDAY	
5K TIME	FES 7 TEMPO	FES 6 TEMPO	FES 5 TEMPO	FES 5 LONG	FES 4 LONG
28:00	09:17	09:33	09:49	10:07	10:18
28:10	09:20	09:36	09:52	10:10	10:21
28:20	09:23	09:39	09:55	10:13	10:24
28:30	09:26	09:42	09:59	10:16	10:28
28:40	09:30	09:46	10:02	10:19	10:31
28:50	09:33	09:49	10:05	10:23	10:34
29:00	09:36	09:52	10:08	10:26	10:37
29:10	09:39	09:55	10:11	10:29	10:40
29:20	09:42	09:59	10:15	10:32	10:44
29:30	09:46	10:02	10:18	10:36	10:47
29:40	09:49	10:05	10:21	10:39	10:50
29:50	09:52	10:08	10:24	10:42	10:53
30:00	09:55	10:11	10:28	10:45	10:56
30:10	09:59	10:15	10:31	10:48	11:00
30:20	10:02	10:18	10:34	10:52	11:03
30:30	10:05	10:21	10:37	10:55	11:06
30:40	10:08	10:24	10:40	10:58	11:09
30:50	10:11	10:28	10:44	11:01	11:13
31:00	10:15	10:31	10:47	11:05	11:16
31:10	10:18	10:34	10:50	11:08	11:19
31:20	10:21	10:37	10:53	11:11	11:22
31:30	10:24	10:40	10:56	11:14	11:25
31:40	10:28	10:44	11:00	11:17	11:29
31:50	10:31	10:47	11:03	11:21	11:32
32:00	10:34	10:50	11:06	11:24	11:35
32:10	10:37	10:53	11:09	11:27	11:38
32:20	10:40	10:56	11:13	11:30	11:42
32:30	10:44	11:00	11:16	11:33	11:45
32:40	10:47	11:03	11:19	11:37	11:48
32:50	10:50	11:06	11:22	11:40	11:51
33:00	10:53	11:09	11:25	11:43	11:54
33:10	10:56	11:13	11:29	11:46	11:58
33:20	11:00	11:16	11:32	11:50	12:01
33:30	11:03	11:19	11:35	11:53	12:04
33:40	11:06	11:22	11:38	11:56	12:07
33:50	11:09	11:25	11:42	11:59	12:10
34:00	11:13	11:29	11:45	12:02	12:14

Minutes per Mile

	TUESDAY		
5K TIME	2 MIN. @	3 MIN. @	5 MIN.@
34:10	10:19	10:31	10:39
34:20	10:23	10:34	10:42
34:30	10:26	10:37	10:45
34:40	10:29	10:40	10:48
34:50	10:32	10:44	10:52
35:00	10:36	10:47	10:55
35:10	10:39	10:50	10:58
35:20	10:42	10:53	11:01
35:30	10:45	10:56	11:05
35:40	10:48	11:00	11:08
35:50	10:52	11:03	11:11
36:00	10:55	11:06	11:14
36:10	10:58	11:09	11:17
36:20	11:01	11:13	11:21
36:30	11:05	11:16	11:24
36:40	11:08	11:19	11:27
36:50	11:11	11:22	11:30
37:00	11:14	11:25	11:33
37:10	11:17	11:29	11:37
37:20	11:21	11:32	11:40
37:30	11:24	11:35	11:43
37:40	11:27	11:38	11:46
37:50	11:30	11:42	11:50
38:00	11:33	11:45	11:53
38:10	11:37	11:48	11:56
38:20	11:40	11:51	11:59
38:30	11:43	11:54	12:02
38:40	11:46	11:58	12:06
38:50	11:50	12:01	12:09
39:00	11:53	12:04	12:12
39:10	11:56	12:07	12:15
39:20	11:59	12:10	12:19
39:30	12:02	12:14	12:22
39:40	12:06	12:17	12:25
39:50	12:09	12:20	12:28
40:00	12:12	12:23	12:31

5K TIME	THURSDAY			SATURDAY	
	FES 7 TEMPO	FES 6 TEMPO	FES 5 TEMPO	FES 5 LONG	FES 4 LONG
34:10	11:16	11:32	11:48	12:06	12:17
34:20	11:19	11:35	11:51	12:09	12:20
34:30	11:22	11:38	11:54	12:12	12:23
34:40	11:25	11:42	11:58	12:15	12:27
34:50	11:29	11:45	12:01	12:19	12:30
35:00	11:32	11:48	12:04	12:22	12:33
35:10	11:35	11:51	12:07	12:25	12:36
35:20	11:38	11:54	12:10	12:28	12:39
35:30	11:42	11:58	12:14	12:31	12:43
35:40	11:45	12:01	12:17	12:35	12:46
35:50	11:48	12:04	12:20	12:38	12:49
36:00	11:51	12:07	12:23	12:41	12:52
36:10	11:54	12:10	12:27	12:44	12:56
36:20	11:58	12:14	12:30	12:47	12:59
36:30	12:01	12:17	12:33	12:51	13:02
36:40	12:04	12:20	12:36	12:54	13:05
36:50	12:07	12:23	12:39	12:57	13:08
37:00	12:10	12:27	12:43	13:00	13:12
37:10	12:14	12:30	12:46	13:04	13:15
37:20	12:17	12:33	12:49	13:07	13:18
37:30	12:20	12:36	12:52	13:10	13:21
37:40	12:23	12:39	12:56	13:13	13:25
37:50	12:27	12:43	12:59	13:16	13:28
38:00	12:30	12:46	13:02	13:20	13:31
38:10	12:33	12:49	13:05	13:23	13:34
38:20	12:36	12:52	13:08	13:26	13:37
38:30	12:39	12:56	13:12	13:29	13:41
38:40	12:43	12:59	13:15	13:33	13:44
38:50	12:46	13:02	13:18	13:36	13:47
39:00	12:49	13:05	13:21	13:39	13:50
39:10	12:52	13:08	13:25	13:42	13:53
39:20	12:56	13:12	13:28	13:45	13:57
39:30	12:59	13:15	13:31	13:49	14:00
39:40	13:02	13:18	13:34	13:52	14:03
39:50	13:05	13:21	13:37	13:55	14:06
40:00	13:08	13:25	13:41	13:58	14:10

Minutes per Kilometer

5K TIME	TUESDAY		
	2 MIN. @	3 MIN. @	5 MIN.@
16:00	02:47	02:54	02:59
16:10	02:49	02:56	03:01
16:20	02:51	02:58	03:03
16:30	02:53	03:00	03:05
16:40	02:55	03:02	03:07
16:50	02:57	03:04	03:09
17:00	02:59	03:06	03:11
17:10	03:01	03:08	03:13
17:20	03:03	03:10	03:15
17:30	03:05	03:12	03:17
17:40	03:07	03:14	03:19
17:50	03:09	03:16	03:21
18:00	03:11	03:18	03:23
18:10	03:13	03:20	03:25
18:20	03:15	03:22	03:27
18:30	03:17	03:24	03:29
18:40	03:19	03:26	03:31
18:50	03:21	03:28	03:33
19:00	03:23	03:30	03:35
19:10	03:25	03:32	03:37
19:20	03:27	03:34	03:39
19:30	03:29	03:36	03:41
19:40	03:31	03:38	03:43
19:50	03:33	03:40	03:45
20:00	03:35	03:42	03:47
20:10	03:37	03:44	03:49
20:20	03:39	03:46	03:51
20:30	03:41	03:48	03:53
20:40	03:43	03:50	03:55
20:50	03:45	03:52	03:57
21:00	03:47	03:54	03:59
21:10	03:49	03:56	04:01
21:20	03:51	03:58	04:03
21:30	03:53	04:00	04:05
21:40	03:55	04:02	04:07

5K TIME	THURSDAY			SATURDAY	
	FES 7 TEMPO	FES 6 TEMPO	FES 5 TEMPO	FES 5 LONG	FES 4 LONG
16:00	03:22	03:32	03:42	03:53	04:00
16:10	03:24	03:34	03:44	03:55	04:02
16:20	03:26	03:36	03:46	03:57	04:04
16:30	03:28	03:38	03:48	03:59	04:06
16:40	03:30	03:40	03:50	04:01	04:08
16:50	03:32	03:42	03:52	04:03	04:10
17:00	03:34	03:44	03:54	04:05	04:12
17:10	03:36	03:46	03:56	04:07	04:14
17:20	03:38	03:48	03:58	04:09	04:16
17:30	03:40	03:50	04:00	04:11	04:18
17:40	03:42	03:52	04:02	04:13	04:20
17:50	03:44	03:54	04:04	04:15	04:22
18:00	03:46	03:56	04:06	04:17	04:24
18:10	03:48	03:58	04:08	04:19	04:26
18:20	03:50	04:00	04:10	04:21	04:28
18:30	03:52	04:02	04:12	04:23	04:30
18:40	03:54	04:04	04:14	04:25	04:32
18:50	03:56	04:06	04:16	04:27	04:34
19:00	03:58	04:08	04:18	04:29	04:36
19:10	04:00	04:10	04:20	04:31	04:38
19:20	04:02	04:12	04:22	04:33	04:40
19:30	04:04	04:14	04:24	04:35	04:42
19:40	04:06	04:16	04:26	04:37	04:44
19:50	04:08	04:18	04:28	04:39	04:46
20:00	04:10	04:20	04:30	04:41	04:48
20:10	04:12	04:22	04:32	04:43	04:50
20:20	04:14	04:24	04:34	04:45	04:52
20:30	04:16	04:26	04:36	04:47	04:54
20:40	04:18	04:28	04:38	04:49	04:56
20:50	04:20	04:30	04:40	04:51	04:58
21:00	04:22	04:32	04:42	04:53	05:00
21:10	04:24	04:34	04:44	04:55	05:02
21:20	04:26	04:36	04:46	04:57	05:04
21:30	04:28	04:38	04:48	04:59	05:06
21:40	04:30	04:40	04:50	05:01	05:08

Minutes per Kilometer

5K TIME	TUESDAY		
	2 MIN. @	3 MIN. @	5 MIN.@
21:50	03:57	04:04	04:09
22:00	03:59	04:06	04:11
22:10	04:01	04:08	04:13
22:20	04:03	04:10	04:15
22:30	04:05	04:12	04:17
22:40	04:07	04:14	04:19
22:50	04:09	04:16	04:21
23:00	04:11	04:18	04:23
23:10	04:13	04:20	04:25
23:20	04:15	04:22	04:27
23:30	04:17	04:24	04:29
23:40	04:19	04:26	04:31
23:50	04:21	04:28	04:33
24:00	04:23	04:30	04:35
24:10	04:25	04:32	04:37
24:20	04:27	04:34	04:39
24:30	04:29	04:36	04:41
24:40	04:31	04:38	04:43
24:50	04:33	04:40	04:45
25:00	04:35	04:42	04:47
25:10	04:37	04:44	04:49
25:20	04:39	04:46	04:51
25:30	04:41	04:48	04:53
25:40	04:43	04:50	04:55
25:50	04:45	04:52	04:57
26:00	04:47	04:54	04:59
26:10	04:49	04:56	05:01
26:20	04:51	04:58	05:03
26:30	04:53	05:00	05:05
26:40	04:55	05:02	05:07
26:50	04:57	05:04	05:09
27:00	04:59	05:06	05:11
27:10	05:01	05:08	05:13
27:20	05:03	05:10	05:15
27:30	05:05	05:12	05:17
27:40	05:07	05:14	05:19
27:50	05:09	05:16	05:21

5K TIME	THURSDAY			SATURDAY	
	FES 7 TEMPO	FES 6 TEMPO	FES 5 TEMPO	FES 5 LONG	FES 4 LONG
21:50	04:32	04:42	04:52	05:03	05:10
22:00	04:34	04:44	04:54	05:05	05:12
22:10	04:36	04:46	04:56	05:07	05:14
22:20	04:38	04:48	04:58	05:09	05:16
22:30	04:40	04:50	05:00	05:11	05:18
22:40	04:42	04:52	05:02	05:13	05:20
22:50	04:44	04:54	05:04	05:15	05:22
23:00	04:46	04:56	05:06	05:17	05:24
23:10	04:48	04:58	05:08	05:19	05:26
23:20	04:50	05:00	05:10	05:21	05:28
23:30	04:52	05:02	05:12	05:23	05:30
23:40	04:54	05:04	05:14	05:25	05:32
23:50	04:56	05:06	05:16	05:27	05:34
24:00	04:58	05:08	05:18	05:29	05:36
24:10	05:00	05:10	05:20	05:31	05:38
24:20	05:02	05:12	05:22	05:33	05:40
24:30	05:04	05:14	05:24	05:35	05:42
24:40	05:06	05:16	05:26	05:37	05:44
24:50	05:08	05:18	05:28	05:39	05:46
25:00	05:10	05:20	05:30	05:41	05:48
25:10	05:12	05:22	05:32	05:43	05:50
25:20	05:14	05:24	05:34	05:45	05:52
25:30	05:16	05:26	05:36	05:47	05:54
25:40	05:18	05:28	05:38	05:49	05:56
25:50	05:20	05:30	05:40	05:51	05:58
26:00	05:22	05:32	05:42	05:53	06:00
26:10	05:24	05:34	05:44	05:55	06:02
26:20	05:26	05:36	05:46	05:57	06:04
26:30	05:28	05:38	05:48	05:59	06:06
26:40	05:30	05:40	05:50	06:01	06:08
26:50	05:32	05:42	05:52	06:03	06:10
27:00	05:34	05:44	05:54	06:05	06:12
27:10	05:36	05:46	05:56	06:07	06:14
27:20	05:38	05:48	05:58	06:09	06:16
27:30	05:40	05:50	06:00	06:11	06:18
27:40	05:42	05:52	06:02	06:13	06:20
27:50	05:44	05:54	06:04	06:15	06:22

Minutes per Kilometer

	TUESDAY		
5K TIME	2 MIN. @	3 MIN. @	5 MIN.@
28:00	05:11	05:18	05:23
28:10	05:13	05:20	05:25
28:20	05:15	05:22	05:27
28:30	05:17	05:24	05:29
28:40	05:19	05:26	05:31
28:50	05:21	05:28	05:33
29:00	05:23	05:30	05:35
29:10	05:25	05:32	05:37
29:20	05:27	05:34	05:39
29:30	05:29	05:36	05:41
29:40	05:31	05:38	05:43
29:50	05:33	05:40	05:45
30:00	05:35	05:42	05:47
30:10	05:37	05:44	05:49
30:20	05:39	05:46	05:51
30:30	05:41	05:48	05:53
30:40	05:43	05:50	05:55
30:50	05:45	05:52	05:57
31:00	05:47	05:54	05:59
31:10	05:49	05:56	06:01
31:20	05:51	05:58	06:03
31:30	05:53	06:00	06:05
31:40	05:55	06:02	06:07
31:50	05:57	06:04	06:09
32:00	05:59	06:06	06:11
32:10	06:01	06:08	06:13
32:20	06:03	06:10	06:15
32:30	06:05	06:12	06:17
32:40	06:07	06:14	06:19
32:50	06:09	06:16	06:21
33:00	06:11	06:18	06:23
33:10	06:13	06:20	06:25
33:20	06:15	06:22	06:27
33:30	06:17	06:24	06:29
33:40	06:19	06:26	06:31
33:50	06:21	06:28	06:33
34:00	06:23	06:30	06:35
34:10	06:25	06:32	06:37

	THURSDAY			SATURDAY	
5K TIME	FES 7 TEMPO	FES 6 TEMPO	FES 5 TEMPO	FES 5 LONG	FES 4 LONG
28:00	05:46	05:56	06:06	06:17	06:24
28:10	05:48	05:58	06:08	06:19	06:26
28:20	05:50	06:00	06:10	06:21	06:28
28:30	05:52	06:02	06:12	06:23	06:30
28:40	05:54	06:04	06:14	06:25	06:32
28:50	05:56	06:06	06:16	06:27	06:34
29:00	05:58	06:08	06:18	06:29	06:36
29:10	06:00	06:10	06:20	06:31	06:38
29:20	06:02	06:12	06:22	06:33	06:40
29:30	06:04	06:14	06:24	06:35	06:42
29:40	06:06	06:16	06:26	06:37	06:44
29:50	06:08	06:18	06:28	06:39	06:46
30:00	06:10	06:20	06:30	06:41	06:48
30:10	06:12	06:22	06:32	06:43	06:50
30:20	06:14	06:24	06:34	06:45	06:52
30:30	06:16	06:26	06:36	06:47	06:54
30:40	06:18	06:28	06:38	06:49	06:56
30:50	06:20	06:30	06:40	06:51	06:58
31:00	06:22	06:32	06:42	06:53	07:00
31:10	06:24	06:34	06:44	06:55	07:02
31:20	06:26	06:36	06:46	06:57	07:04
31:30	06:28	06:38	06:48	06:59	07:06
31:40	06:30	06:40	06:50	07:01	07:08
31:50	06:32	06:42	06:52	07:03	07:10
32:00	06:34	06:44	06:54	07:05	07:12
32:10	06:36	06:46	06:56	07:07	07:14
32:20	06:38	06:48	06:58	07:09	07:16
32:30	06:40	06:50	07:00	07:11	07:18
32:40	06:42	06:52	07:02	07:13	07:20
32:50	06:44	06:54	07:04	07:15	07:22
33:00	06:46	06:56	07:06	07:17	07:24
33:10	06:48	06:58	07:08	07:19	07:26
33:20	06:50	07:00	07:10	07:21	07:28
33:30	06:52	07:02	07:12	07:23	07:30
33:40	06:54	07:04	07:14	07:25	07:32
33:50	06:56	07:06	07:16	07:27	07:34
34:00	06:58	07:08	07:18	07:29	07:36
34:10	07:00	07:10	07:20	07:31	07:38

Minutes per Kilometer

	TUESDAY		
5K TIME	2 MIN. @	3 MIN. @	5 MIN.@
34:20	06:27	06:34	06:39
34:30	06:29	06:36	06:41
34:40	06:31	06:38	06:43
34:50	06:33	06:40	06:45
35:00	06:35	06:42	06:47
35:10	06:37	06:44	06:49
35:20	06:39	06:46	06:51
35:30	06:41	06:48	06:53
35:40	06:43	06:50	06:55
35:50	06:45	06:52	06:57
36:00	06:47	06:54	06:59
36:10	06:49	06:56	07:01
36:20	06:51	06:58	07:03
36:30	06:53	07:00	07:05
36:40	06:55	07:02	07:07
36:50	06:57	07:04	07:09
37:00	06:59	07:06	07:11
37:10	07:01	07:08	07:13
37:20	07:03	07:10	07:15
37:30	07:05	07:12	07:17
37:40	07:07	07:14	07:19
37:50	07:09	07:16	07:21
38:00	07:11	07:18	07:23
38:10	07:13	07:20	07:25
38:20	07:15	07:22	07:27
38:30	07:17	07:24	07:29
38:40	07:19	07:26	07:31
38:50	07:21	07:28	07:33
39:00	07:23	07:30	07:35
39:10	07:25	07:32	07:37
39:20	07:27	07:34	07:39
39:30	07:29	07:36	07:41
39:40	07:31	07:38	07:43
39:50	07:33	07:40	07:45
40:00	07:35	07:42	07:47

	THURSDAY			SATURDAY	
5K TIME	FES 7 TEMPO	FES 6 TEMPO	FES 5 TEMPO	FES 5 LONG	FES 4 LONG
34:20	07:02	07:12	07:22	07:33	07:40
34:30	07:04	07:14	07:24	07:35	07:42
34:40	07:06	07:16	07:26	07:37	07:44
34:50	07:08	07:18	07:28	07:39	07:46
35:00	07:10	07:20	07:30	07:41	07:48
35:10	07:12	07:22	07:32	07:43	07:50
35:20	07:14	07:24	07:34	07:45	07:52
35:30	07:16	07:26	07:36	07:47	07:54
35:40	07:18	07:28	07:38	07:49	07:56
35:50	07:20	07:30	07:40	07:51	07:58
36:00	07:22	07:32	07:42	07:53	08:00
36:10	07:24	07:34	07:44	07:55	08:02
36:20	07:26	07:36	07:46	07:57	08:04
36:30	07:28	07:38	07:48	07:59	08:06
36:40	07:30	07:40	07:50	08:01	08:08
36:50	07:32	07:42	07:52	08:03	08:10
37:00	07:34	07:44	07:54	08:05	08:12
37:10	07:36	07:46	07:56	08:07	08:14
37:20	07:38	07:48	07:58	08:09	08:16
37:30	07:40	07:50	08:00	08:11	08:18
37:40	07:42	07:52	08:02	08:13	08:20
37:50	07:44	07:54	08:04	08:15	08:22
38:00	07:46	07:56	08:06	08:17	08:24
38:10	07:48	07:58	08:08	08:19	08:26
38:20	07:50	08:00	08:10	08:21	08:28
38:30	07:52	08:02	08:12	08:23	08:30
38:40	07:54	08:04	08:14	08:25	08:32
38:50	07:56	08:06	08:16	08:27	08:34
39:00	07:58	08:08	08:18	08:29	08:36
39:10	08:00	08:10	08:20	08:31	08:38
39:20	08:02	08:12	08:22	08:33	08:40
39:30	08:04	08:14	08:24	08:35	08:42
39:40	08:06	08:16	08:26	08:37	08:44
39:50	08:08	08:18	08:28	08:39	08:46
40:00	08:10	08:20	08:30	08:41	08:48

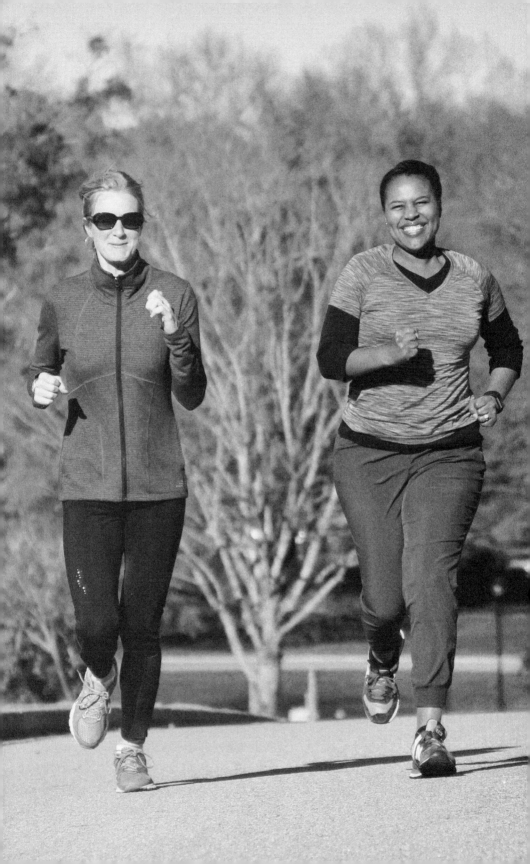

APPENDIX B

SUPPLEMENTAL WORKOUTS

CYCLING

HIGH-INTENSITY THRESHOLD WORKOUT (30 MINUTES)

- 10 minutes at FES of 2.
- 5 minutes at FES of 5.
- 5 minutes at FES of 6.
- 5 minutes at FES of 7.
- 5 minutes at FES of 2 as a cooldown.

HIGH-INTENSITY INTERVAL WORKOUT (30 MINUTES)

- 3 minutes of cycling at FES of 2.
- 5 x (3 minutes increased resistance at FES of 6, 2 minutes at FES of 2).
- 2 more minutes at FES of 2 as a cooldown.

HIGH-CADENCE THRESHOLD WORKOUT (30 MINUTES)

- 5 minutes of cycling at FES of 2.
- 10 minutes of fast cycling at FES of 5.
- 5 minutes at FES of 3.
- 5 min at FES of 7.
- 5 minutes at FES of 2 as a cooldown.

OVER/UNDER WORKOUT (30 MINUTES)

- 5 minutes of cycling at FES of 2.
- Check your cadence the last few minutes of the warmup.
- Continue for 4 minutes at a cadence that is 12 rpm faster than your warmup cadence.
- You might not need to adjust the resistance.
- Next do 3 minutes at a cadence that is 12 rpm slower than your warmup cadence.
- You will need to increase the resistance.

- Alternate this over/under cadence sequence two more times.
- 4 minutes at FES of 2 as a cooldown.

FAST LEG TURNOVER WORKOUT (30 MINUTES)

- 5 minutes of cycling at FES of 2.
  Keep the resistance the same and relatively light for 10 sequences of . . .
- 10 x (alternate 1 minute of fast cycling at FES of 7, 1 minute at FES of 2).
- 5 minutes at FES of 2 as a cooldown.

THRESHOLD/INTENSITY WORKOUT (30 MINUTES)

- 5 minutes of cycling at FES of 2.
- 15 minutes at FES of 6.
- 2 minutes at FES of 2.
- 3 x (1 minute at FES of 7, 1 minute at FES of 2).
- 2 minutes at FES of 2 as a cooldown.

RUNNING

TUESDAY SPEED RUN WORKOUT (48 MINUTES*)

- 5 minutes at FES of 2 progressing to FES of 3 as a warmup.
- 4 minutes fast at FES of 7, followed by a recovery of 1 minute at FES of 2.
- 4 x (1 minute fast at FES of 8), followed by a recovery of 1 minute at FES of 2.
- 3 x (2 minutes fast at FES of 7), followed by a recovery of 1 minute at FES of 2.
- 2 x (3 minutes fast at FES of 8), followed by a recovery of 1 minute at FES of 2.
- 4 x (1 minute fast at FES of 7).
- 5 minutes at FES of 2 as a cooldown.

*Total fast running of 24 minutes

THURSDAY TEMPO RUN WORKOUT (45 MINUTES)

- First 10 minutes at FES of 2–3.
- 10 minutes at FES of 5.
- 10 minutes a little faster at FES of 6.
- Final 10 minutes at FES of 7–8.
- 5 minutes at FES of 2 as a cooldown.

THURSDAY TEMPO RUN WORKOUT (40 MINUTES)

- First 10 minutes at FES of 2–3.
- 10 minutes at FES of 7.
- 5 minutes at FES of 2–3.
- 10 minutes at FES of 7–8.
- 5 minutes at FES at 2 as a cooldown.

ROWING

TEMPO/THRESHOLD WORKOUT (23–25 MINUTES)

- 4 minutes at FES of 2–3 as a warmup.
- 3 x (1000 meters at FES of 8; rest for 90 seconds between efforts).
- 4 minutes at FES of 2–3 as a cooldown.

HIGH-INTENSITY INTERVAL WORKOUT (25 MINUTES)

- 5 minutes at FES of 2–3 as a warmup.
- 3 x (1 minute fast at FES of 8, 1 minute rest).
- 2 x (2 minutes fast at FES of 7, 1 minute rest).
- 3 minutes fast at FES of 7.
- 5 minutes at FES of 2 as a cooldown.

ELLIPTICAL TRAINER

MODERATE-INTENSITY INTERVAL WORKOUT (35 MINUTES)

- 5 minutes at FES of 2.
- 5 minutes at FES of 5.
- 5 minutes at FES of 2.
- 5 minutes at FES of 7.
- 5 minutes at FES of 2–3.
- 5 minutes at FES of 5.
- 5 minutes at FES of 2.

MODERATE-INTENSITY, LOW-RESISTANCE INTERVAL WORKOUT (35 MINUTES)

- 4 minutes at FES of 2.
  Keep the resistance the same and relatively light:
- 7 x (alternate 2 minutes fast at FES of 5 and 2 minutes at FES of 2).
- 3 minutes at FES of 2 as a cooldown.

MODERATE-INTENSITY, LOW-RESISTANCE INTERVAL WORKOUT (35 MINUTES)

- 5 minutes at FES of 2.
  Keep the resistance relatively light:
- 5 x (alternate 3-minute fast stride rate at FES of 5 and 2 minutes at FES of 2–3).
- 5 minutes at FES of 2 as a cooldown.

FAST-CADENCE WORKOUT (35 MINUTES)

- 5 minutes at FES of 2.
- 10 minutes with a fast stride rate at FES of 4.

- 10 minutes with a faster stride rate at FES of 5.
- 2 minutes at FES of 2–3.
- 5 minutes with an increased resistance at FES of 5.
- 3 minutes at FES of 2 as a cooldown.

HIGH-INTENSITY INTERVAL WORKOUT (35 MINUTES)

- 10 minutes at FES of 2.
- 5 minutes at FES of 5.
- 3 minutes at FES of 2–3.
- 3 x (2 minutes at FES of 6, 2 minutes at FES of 2).
- 5 minutes at FES of 2 as a cooldown.

APPENDIX C

How to Convert Your Current Time to an Equivalent Time at an Earlier Age

FIND THE AGE-ADJUSTMENT FACTOR FOR your age and race distance in the Road Age Factors WMA 2015 table for your sex in the following tables. Multiply that age factor by your current race time to determine your equivalent race time at your prime-age time.

For example, a 60-year-old male whose time for the 5-K is 20:00 minutes would multiply that time by the age factor of 0.8131 and see that it is equivalent to a 16:15 at the prime 5-K performance age for males, the 22- to 28-year-old age group.

A 50-year-old female whose time for the marathon is 4:00:00 would multiply that 4:00:00 by the age factor of 0.8796 and see that it is equivalent to a 3:31:06 at the prime marathon performance age for females, which is at approximately age 30.

Road Age Factors

		Male		
AGE	5-K	10-K	HALF-MARATHON	MARATHON
30	0.9970	1.0000	1.0000	1.0000
31	0.9947	0.9996	1.0000	1.0000
32	0.9918	0.9984	0.9998	0.9998
33	0.9882	0.9966	0.9989	0.9989
34	0.9839	0.9941	0.9973	0.9973
35	0.9790	0.9908	0.9950	0.9950
36	0.9734	0.9869	0.9920	0.9920
37	0.9672	0.9822	0.9882	0.9882
38	0.9605	0.9769	0.9837	0.9837
39	0.9538	0.9708	0.9784	0.9784
40	0.9471	0.9640	0.9725	0.9725
41	0.9404	0.9566	0.9658	0.9658
42	0.9337	0.9491	0.9584	0.9584
43	0.9270	0.9417	0.9506	0.9506
44	0.9203	0.9342	0.9428	0.9428
45	0.9136	0.9267	0.9350	0.9350
46	0.9069	0.9192	0.9273	0.9273
47	0.9002	0.9117	0.9195	0.9195
48	0.8935	0.9043	0.9117	0.9117
49	0.8868	0.8968	0.9039	0.9039
50	0.8801	0.8893	0.8961	0.8961
51	0.8734	0.8818	0.8884	0.8884
52	0.8667	0.8743	0.8806	0.8806
53	0.8600	0.8669	0.8728	0.8728

Female				
AGE	5-K	10-K	HALF-MARATHON	MARATHON
30	1.0000	1.0000	0.9997	1.0000
31	0.9998	0.9998	0.9989	0.9998
32	0.9990	0.9989	0.9975	0.9989
33	0.9977	0.9975	0.9956	0.9974
34	0.9959	0.9955	0.9931	0.9953
35	0.9935	0.9930	0.9901	0.9926
36	0.9906	0.9898	0.9865	0.9893
37	0.9871	0.9860	0.9823	0.9854
38	0.9831	0.9817	0.9776	0.9808
39	0.9785	0.9768	0.9724	0.9757
40	0.9734	0.9713	0.9666	0.9699
41	0.9678	0.9652	0.9602	0.9635
42	0.9616	0.9585	0.9533	0.9565
43	0.9549	0.9512	0.9458	0.9489
44	0.9476	0.9433	0.9378	0.9406
45	0.9398	0.9349	0.9293	0.9318
46	0.9314	0.9259	0.9201	0.9223
47	0.9225	0.9162	0.9105	0.9122
48	0.9131	0.9060	0.9003	0.9016
49	0.9034	0.8955	0.8898	0.8906
50	0.8937	0.8850	0.8793	0.8796
51	0.8840	0.8745	0.8688	0.8686
52	0.8743	0.8640	0.8583	0.8576
53	0.8645	0.8535	0.8478	0.8466

Male				
AGE	5-K	10-K	HALF-MARATHON	MARATHON
54	0.8533	0.8594	0.8650	0.8650
55	0.8466	0.8519	0.8572	0.8572
56	0.8399	0.8444	0.8495	0.8495
57	0.8332	0.8369	0.8417	0.8417
58	0.8265	0.8295	0.8339	0.8339
59	0.8198	0.8220	0.8261	0.8261
60	0.8131	0.8145	0.8183	0.8183
61	0.8064	0.8070	0.8106	0.8106
62	0.7997	0.7995	0.8028	0.8028
63	0.7930	0.7921	0.7950	0.7950
64	0.7863	0.7846	0.7872	0.7872
65	0.7796	0.7771	0.7794	0.7794
66	0.7729	0.7696	0.7717	0.7717
67	0.7662	0.7621	0.7639	0.7639
68	0.7592	0.7547	0.7561	0.7561
69	0.7515	0.7471	0.7483	0.7483
70	0.7433	0.7391	0.7405	0.7405
71	0.7344	0.7305	0.7324	0.7324
72	0.7249	0.7211	0.7236	0.7236
73	0.7147	0.7112	0.7140	0.7140
74	0.7040	0.7005	0.7038	0.7038
75	0.6926	0.6892	0.6929	0.6929
76	0.6806	0.6772	0.6813	0.6813
77	0.6680	0.6646	0.6689	0.6689
78	0.6547	0.6513	0.6559	0.6559

Female				
AGE	5-K	10-K	HALF-MARATHON	MARATHON
54	0.8548	0.8430	0.8373	0.8356
55	0.8451	0.8325	0.8268	0.8246
56	0.8354	0.8220	0.8163	0.8136
57	0.8257	0.8115	0.8058	0.8026
58	0.8160	0.8010	0.7953	0.7916
59	0.8063	0.7905	0.7848	0.7806
60	0.7966	0.7800	0.7743	0.7696
61	0.7869	0.7695	0.7638	0.7586
62	0.7772	0.7590	0.7533	0.7476
63	0.7674	0.7485	0.7428	0.7366
64	0.7577	0.7380	0.7323	0.7256
65	0.7480	0.7275	0.7218	0.7146
66	0.7383	0.7170	0.7113	0.7036
67	0.7286	0.7065	0.7008	0.6926
68	0.7189	0.6960	0.6903	0.6816
69	0.7092	0.6855	0.6798	0.6706
70	0.6995	0.6750	0.6693	0.6596
71	0.6898	0.6645	0.6588	0.6486
72	0.6801	0.6540	0.6483	0.6376
73	0.6703	0.6435	0.6378	0.6266
74	0.6606	0.6330	0.6273	0.6156
75	0.6509	0.6225	0.6168	0.6042
76	0.6412	0.6120	0.6059	0.5920
77	0.6315	0.6015	0.5942	0.5790
78	0.6218	0.5910	0.5818	0.5652

Male				
AGE	5-K	10-K	HALF-MARATHON	MARATHON
79	0.6408	0.6374	0.6422	0.6422
80	0.6263	0.6228	0.6277	0.6277
81	0.6112	0.6075	0.6126	0.6126
82	0.5955	0.5916	0.5968	0.5968
83	0.5791	0.5750	0.5802	0.5802
84	0.5621	0.5577	0.5630	0.5630
85	0.5445	0.5398	0.5451	0.5451
86	0.5262	0.5213	0.5265	0.5265
87	0.5074	0.5020	0.5071	0.5071
88	0.4879	0.4821	0.4871	0.4871
89	0.4678	0.4616	0.4664	0.4664
90	0.4470	0.4404	0.4449	0.4449
91	0.4257	0.4185	0.4228	0.4228
92	0.4037	0.3960	0.4000	0.4000
93	0.3811	0.3728	0.3764	0.3764
94	0.3578	0.3489	0.3522	0.3522
95	0.3340	0.3244	0.3273	0.3273
96	0.3095	0.2993	0.3017	0.3017
97	0.2844	0.2734	0.2753	0.2753
98	0.2586	0.2470	0.2483	0.2483
99	0.2323	0.2198	0.2206	0.2206
100	0.2053	0.1920	0.1921	0.1921

		Female		
AGE	5-K	10-K	HALF-MARATHON	MARATHON
79	0.6120	0.5801	0.5687	0.5506
80	0.6013	0.5681	0.5548	0.5352
81	0.5897	0.5553	0.5401	0.5190
82	0.5772	0.5415	0.5246	0.5020
83	0.5637	0.5268	0.5084	0.4842
84	0.5493	0.5111	0.4915	0.4656
85	0.5340	0.4945	0.4738	0.4462
86	0.5177	0.4769	0.4553	0.4260
87	0.5004	0.4585	0.4360	0.4050
88	0.4823	0.4390	0.4160	0.3832
89	0.4632	0.4187	0.3953	0.3606
90	0.4431	0.3973	0.3738	0.3372
91	0.4221	0.3751	0.3515	0.3130
92	0.4002	0.3519	0.3284	0.2880
93	0.3773	0.3278	0.3046	0.2622
94	0.3535	0.3027	0.2801	0.2356
95	0.3288	0.2767	0.2548	0.2082
96	0.3031	0.2497	0.2287	0.1800
97	0.2764	0.2219	0.2018	0.1510
98	0.2489	0.1930	0.1742	0.1212
99	0.2204	0.1633	0.1459	0.0906
100	0.1909	0.1325	0.1168	0.0592

Approved by the WMA and USATF
Compiled by Alan Jones with Rex Harvey
AlanLJones@stny.rr.com
http://runscore.com/Alan/AgeGrade.html

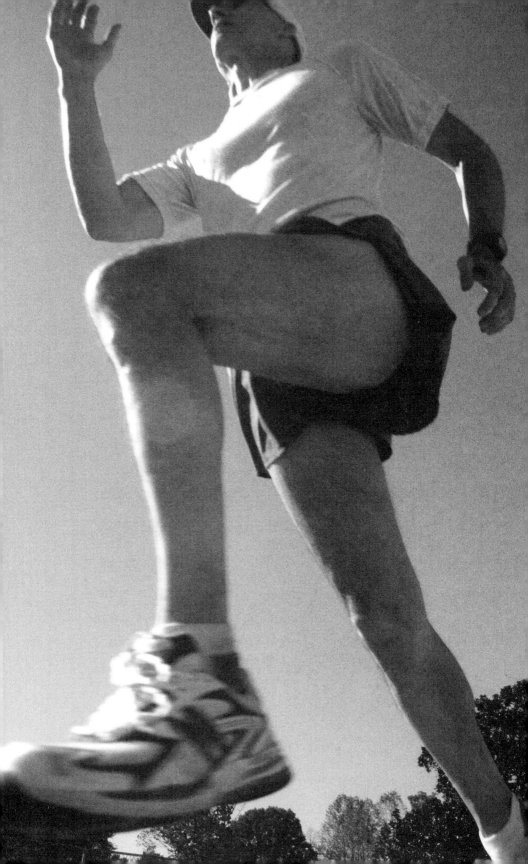

APPENDIX D

How to Compare Your Current Time to the World-Class Time for Your Age

FIND THE WORLD-CLASS TIME FOR your age and race distance in the Road Age Standards WMA 2015 table for your sex in the following tables. Divide your current time by the world-class race time for your age to determine your performance level percentage (PLP) of world-class time.

For example, a 60-year-old male whose time for the 5-K is 20:20 minutes (20.333 minutes) would divide 20.333 into the world-class time of 15:58 minutes (15.97 minutes) and see that he is running at a PLP of 78.5 percent of world-class time for his age.

A 50-year-old female whose time for the marathon is 4:01:30 (241.5 minutes) would divide 241.5 into the world-class time of 2:33:57 (153.95 minutes) and see that she is running at a PLP of 63.7 percent of world-class time for her age.

Performance Level Percentage Categories

- 100 percent = World Record Level
- 90 to 99 percent = World Class
- 80 to 89 percent = National Class

- 70 to 79 percent = Regional Class
- 60 to 69 percent = Local Class

Road Age Standards

		Male		
AGE	5-K	10-K	HALF-MARATHON	MARATHON
30	0:13:01	0:26:43	0:58:23	2:02:57
31	0:13:03	0:26:44	0:58:23	2:02:57
32	0:13:05	0:26:46	0:58:24	2:02:58
33	0:13:08	0:26:48	0:58:27	2:03:05
34	0:13:12	0:26:53	0:58:32	2:03:17
35	0:13:16	0:26:58	0:58:41	2:03:34
36	0:13:20	0:27:04	0:58:51	2:03:56
37	0:13:25	0:27:12	0:59:05	2:04:25
38	0:13:31	0:27:21	0:59:21	2:04:59
39	0:13:37	0:27:31	0:59:40	2:05:40
40	0:13:43	0:27:43	1:00:02	2:06:26
41	0:13:48	0:27:56	1:00:27	2:07:18
42	0:13:54	0:28:09	1:00:55	2:08:17
43	0:14:00	0:28:22	1:01:25	2:09:20
44	0:14:06	0:28:36	1:01:56	2:10:25
45	0:14:13	0:28:50	1:02:27	2:11:30
46	0:14:19	0:29:04	1:02:58	2:12:35
47	0:14:25	0:29:18	1:03:30	2:13:43
48	0:14:32	0:29:33	1:04:02	2:14:51
49	0:14:38	0:29:47	1:04:35	2:16:01
50	0:14:45	0:30:03	1:05:09	2:17:12

	Female			
AGE	5-K	10-K	HALF-MARATHON	MARATHON
30	0:14:46	0:30:20	1:05:13	2:15:25
31	0:14:46	0:30:20	1:05:16	2:15:27
32	0:14:47	0:30:22	1:05:22	2:15:34
33	0:14:48	0:30:25	1:05:29	2:15:46
34	0:14:50	0:30:28	1:05:39	2:16:03
35	0:14:52	0:30:33	1:05:51	2:16:26
36	0:14:54	0:30:39	1:06:06	2:16:53
37	0:14:58	0:30:46	1:06:22	2:17:25
38	0:15:01	0:30:54	1:06:42	2:18:04
39	0:15:05	0:31:03	1:07:03	2:18:47
40	0:15:10	0:31:14	1:07:27	2:19:37
41	0:15:15	0:31:26	1:07:54	2:20:33
42	0:15:21	0:31:39	1:08:24	2:21:35
43	0:15:28	0:31:53	1:08:56	2:22:43
44	0:15:35	0:32:09	1:09:31	2:23:58
45	0:15:43	0:32:27	1:10:10	2:25:20
46	0:15:51	0:32:46	1:10:52	2:26:49
47	0:16:00	0:33:06	1:11:37	2:28:27
48	0:16:10	0:33:29	1:12:25	2:30:12
49	0:16:21	0:33:52	1:13:16	2:32:03
50	0:16:31	0:34:16	1:14:09	2:33:57

Male				
AGE	5-K	10-K	HALF-MARATHON	MARATHON
51	0:14:52	0:30:18	1:05:43	2:18:24
52	0:14:59	0:30:33	1:06:18	2:19:37
53	0:15:06	0:30:49	1:06:54	2:20:52
54	0:15:13	0:31:05	1:07:30	2:22:08
55	0:15:20	0:31:22	1:08:07	2:23:26
56	0:15:27	0:31:38	1:08:44	2:24:44
57	0:15:35	0:31:55	1:09:22	2:26:04
58	0:15:43	0:32:12	1:10:01	2:27:26
59	0:15:50	0:32:30	1:10:40	2:28:50
60	0:15:58	0:32:48	1:11:21	2:30:15
61	0:16:06	0:33:06	1:12:01	2:31:41
62	0:16:14	0:33:25	1:12:43	2:33:09
63	0:16:22	0:33:44	1:13:26	2:34:39
64	0:16:31	0:34:03	1:14:10	2:36:11
65	0:16:39	0:34:23	1:14:54	2:37:45
66	0:16:48	0:34:43	1:15:39	2:39:19
67	0:16:57	0:35:03	1:16:26	2:40:57
68	0:17:06	0:35:24	1:17:13	2:42:37
69	0:17:17	0:35:46	1:18:01	2:44:18
70	0:17:28	0:36:09	1:18:51	2:46:02
71	0:17:41	0:36:34	1:19:43	2:47:52
72	0:17:55	0:37:03	1:20:41	2:49:55
73	0:18:10	0:37:34	1:21:46	2:52:12
74	0:18:27	0:38:08	1:22:57	2:54:42
75	0:18:45	0:38:46	1:24:16	2:57:27
76	0:19:05	0:39:27	1:25:42	3:00:28
77	0:19:26	0:40:12	1:27:17	3:03:49

		Female		
AGE	5-K	10-K	HALF-MARATHON	MARATHON
51	0:16:42	0:34:41	1:15:03	2:35:54
52	0:16:53	0:35:06	1:15:58	2:37:54
53	0:17:05	0:35:32	1:16:54	2:39:57
54	0:17:16	0:35:59	1:17:52	2:42:04
55	0:17:28	0:36:26	1:18:51	2:44:13
56	0:17:41	0:36:54	1:19:52	2:46:26
57	0:17:53	0:37:23	1:20:55	2:48:43
58	0:18:06	0:37:52	1:21:59	2:51:04
59	0:18:19	0:38:22	1:23:05	2:53:29
60	0:18:32	0:38:53	1:24:12	2:55:57
61	0:18:46	0:39:25	1:25:22	2:58:31
62	0:19:00	0:39:58	1:26:33	3:01:08
63	0:19:15	0:40:32	1:27:47	3:03:50
64	0:19:29	0:41:06	1:29:02	3:06:38
65	0:19:44	0:41:42	1:30:20	3:09:30
66	0:20:00	0:42:18	1:31:40	3:12:28
67	0:20:16	0:42:56	1:33:02	3:15:31
68	0:20:32	0:43:35	1:34:27	3:18:40
69	0:20:49	0:44:15	1:35:55	3:21:56
70	0:21:07	0:44:56	1:37:25	3:25:18
71	0:21:24	0:45:39	1:38:58	3:28:47
72	0:21:43	0:46:23	1:40:34	3:32:23
73	0:22:02	0:47:08	1:42:14	3:36:07
74	0:22:21	0:47:55	1:43:56	3:39:59
75	0:22:41	0:48:44	1:45:42	3:44:08
76	0:23:02	0:49:34	1:47:37	3:48:45
77	0:23:23	0:50:26	1:49:44	3:53:53

Male				
AGE	5-K	10-K	HALF-MARATHON	MARATHON
78	0:19:50	0:41:01	1:29:01	3:07:27
79	0:20:16	0:41:55	1:30:55	3:11:27
80	0:20:44	0:42:54	1:33:01	3:15:52
81	0:21:15	0:43:59	1:35:18	3:20:42
82	0:21:48	0:45:10	1:37:50	3:26:01
83	0:22:25	0:46:28	1:40:38	3:31:55
84	0:23:06	0:47:54	1:43:42	3:38:23
85	0:23:51	0:49:30	1:47:06	3:45:33
86	0:24:40	0:51:15	1:50:53	3:53:31
87	0:25:35	0:53:13	1:55:08	4:02:27
88	0:26:37	0:55:25	1:59:52	4:12:25
89	0:27:45	0:57:53	2:05:11	4:23:37
90	0:29:03	1:00:40	2:11:14	4:36:21
91	0:30:30	1:03:50	2:18:05	4:50:48
92	0:32:10	1:07:28	2:25:58	5:07:23
93	0:34:04	1:11:40	2:35:07	5:26:39
94	0:36:17	1:16:34	2:45:46	5:49:05
95	0:38:52	1:22:21	2:58:23	6:15:39
96	0:41:57	1:29:16	3:13:31	6:47:31
97	0:45:39	1:37:43	3:32:04	7:26:36
98	0:50:12	1:48:10	3:55:08	8:15:10
99	0:55:53	2:01:33	4:24:39	9:17:21
100	1:03:14	2:19:09	5:03:55	10:40:02

		Female		
AGE	**5-K**	**10-K**	**HALF-MARATHON**	**MARATHON**
78	0:23:45	0:51:20	1:52:04	3:59:35
79	0:24:08	0:52:17	1:54:39	4:05:57
80	0:24:33	0:53:24	1:57:31	4:13:01
81	0:25:02	0:54:38	2:00:43	4:20:55
82	0:25:35	0:56:01	2:04:17	4:29:45
83	0:26:12	0:57:35	2:08:15	4:39:40
84	0:26:53	0:59:21	2:12:39	4:50:51
85	0:27:39	1:01:20	2:17:37	5:03:29
86	0:28:31	1:03:36	2:23:12	5:17:53
87	0:29:31	1:06:09	2:29:32	5:34:22
88	0:30:37	1:09:06	2:36:44	5:53:23
89	0:31:53	1:12:27	2:44:56	6:15:32
90	0:33:20	1:16:21	2:54:25	6:41:35
91	0:34:59	1:20:52	3:05:29	7:12:38
92	0:36:54	1:26:12	3:18:32	7:50:12
93	0:39:08	1:32:32	3:34:03	8:36:28
94	0:41:46	1:40:13	3:52:46	9:34:46
95	0:44:55	1:49:38	4:15:53	10:50:25
96	0:48:43	2:01:29	4:45:05	12:32:19
97	0:53:25	2:16:42	5:23:06	14:56:48
98	0:59:20	2:37:10	6:14:17	18:37:18
99	1:07:00	3:05:45	7:26:53	24:54:40
100	1:17:21	3:48:56	9:18:13	38:07:27

Approved by the WMA and USATF
Compiled by Alan Jones with Rex Harvey
AlanLJones@stny.rr.com
http://runscore.com/Alan/AgeGrade.html

ACKNOWLEDGMENTS

WE ARE GRATEFUL TO RACHEL TOOR for her offer to review the first draft of our manuscript. Having a published author of multiple books, popular columnist, former Oxford Press editor, and writing professor critique your writing is like having Roger Federer critique your tennis strokes. The feedback might be deflating and painful, but in the end, it makes you better. That's what Rachel's critical edits did for us. We are fortunate that she generously offered her time and expertise to help us convey our message to aging runners.

As with *Runner's World Run Less, Run Faster,* we relied on my brother, Don Pierce, for his thoughts and reactions to all of our ideas, from the first outline of the book to the final draft. He read every word multiple times and participated in all of our discussion sessions as we forged our concepts for the book. His participation as a member of the book's team was essential.

We wish to thank photographer Jeremy Fleming for his time and patience in taking hundreds of photos of our strength training and stretching exercises. His relentless attention to detail gave us the depictions we sought. Similarly, we are grateful to Rita Gary, Furman's cross-country and track-and-field assistant coach, for enduring hours of poses while Jeremy took multiple shots of each exercise. Both brought enthusiasm and stamina to this project.

The encouragement that we received from Mark Weinstein at Rodale led to this book. His support during throughout the process is appreciated. Franny Vignola's prompt and professional editorial support was immensely helpful.

We appreciate Furman University for giving us the opportunity to establish the Furman Institute of Running and Scientific Training. We acknowledge the many runners who, through their messages and participation at the institute, have stimulated our professional careers and enriched our personal lives.

SOURCE NOTES

CHAPTER 1

1. B.R. Londeree, "The Use of Laboratory Test Results with Long Distance Runners," *Sports Medicine* 3, no. 3 (1986): 201–13.

2. W.L. Kenney and J.H. Wilmore, *Physiology of Sport and Exercise*, 5th ed. (Champaign, IL: Human Kinetics, 2011).

3. A.E. Ready and H.A. Quinney, "Alterations in Anaerobic Threshold as the Result of Endurance Training and Detraining," *Medicine and Science in Sports and Exercise* 14, no. 4 (1982): 292–96.

4. V. Billat, "Interval Training at VO$_2$ max: Effects on Aerobic Performance and Overtraining Markers," *Medicine and Science in Sports and Exercise* 31, no. 1 (1999): 156–63.

5. J.E. McLaughlin et al., "Test of the Classic Model for Predicting Endurance Running Performance," *Medicine and Science in Sports and Exercise* 42, no. 5 (2010): 991–97. D.W. Morgan et al., "Ten Kilometer Performance and Predicted Velocity at VO$_2$max among Well-Trained Male Runners," *Medicine and Science in Sports and Exercise* 21, no. 1 (1989): 78–83.

6. B. Mackenzie, "vVO$_2$ max and tlimvVO$_2$ max," BrianMac Sports Coach, https://www.brianmac.co.uk/vvo2max.htm.

7. T.D. Fahey, P.M. Insel, and W.T. Walton, *Fit and Well: Core Concepts and Labs in Physical Fitness and Wellness*, 12th ed. (New York: McGraw-Hill Education, 2017).

CHAPTER 2

1. New York Road Runners, www.nyrr.org.

2. Atlanta Track Club, "2015 AKC Peachtree Road Race," www.atlantatrackclub.org/2015-peachtree.

3. New York Road Runners.

4. J.P. Porcari, C.X. Bryant, and F. Comana, *Exercise Physiology* (Philadelphia: F.A. Davis, 2015).

5. G.W. Heath et al., "A Physiological Comparison of Young and Older Endurance Athletes," *Journal of Applied Physiology* 51, no. 3 (1981): 634–40. S.W. Trappe et al., "Aging among Elite Distance Runners: A 22-Year Longitudinal Study," *Journal of Applied Physiology* 80, no. 1 (1996): 285–90.

6. B. Glover and S. Glover, *The Competitive Runner's Handbook* (New York: Penguin, 1999).

7. R.J. Shepard, "Aging and Exercise," *Encyclopedia of Sports Medicine and Science*, T.D. Fahey, ed. (Internet Society for Sport Science, 1998), http://sportsci.org.

8. T. Noakes, *Lore of Running* (Champaign, IL: Leisure Press, 2001).

9. World Masters Athletics, www.world-masters-athletics.org.

10. National Strength and Conditioning Association, www.nsca.com.

CHAPTER 3

1. Running USA, "Annual Reports," http://www.runningusa.org/annual-reports.

2. San Sebastian (Spain) Marathon, www.maratondonostia.com.
3. Running USA, "Annual Reports."
4. C. Fuller, "For Boston Marathon's Runners, Resolve, and Camaraderie Unshaken," *Christian Science Monitor*, April 22, 2013.
5. L. Crimaldi, "Marathon Runners Raised Record $38.4M for Charity in 2014," *Boston Globe*, July 1, 2014.
6. Fuller, "For Boston Marathon's Runners, Resolve, and Camaraderie Unshaken."
7. Crimaldi, "Marathon Runners Raised Record $38.4M for Charity in 2014."
8. Leukemia & Lymphoma Society Team in Training, www.teamintraining.org.
9. Running USA, "Annual Reports."
10. Ibid.
11. Ibid.
12. New York Road Runners, "History of the New York City Marathon," www.tcsnycmarathon.org/about -the-race/history-of-the-new-york -city-marathon.
13. Rock 'n' Roll Marathon Series, www .runrocknroll.com.
14. R. Toor, "Thirteener Manifesto," *Running Times*, February 27, 2014.
15. 2015 National Runner Survey, Running USA, www.runningusa.org.
16. Ibid.

CHAPTER 4

1. S.C. Mathews et al., "Mortality among Marathon Runners in the United States, 2000–2009," *American Journal of Sports Medicine* 40, no. 7 (2012): 1495–500.
2. T.J. Bassler, "Marathon Running and Immunity to Heart Disease," *Physician Sportsmedicine* 3 (1975): 77–80.
3. J.H. O'Keefe et al., "Potential Adverse Cardiovascular Effects from Excessive Endurance Exercise," *Mayo Clinic Proceedings* 87, no. 6 (2012): 587–95.
4. Physical Activity Guidelines Advisory Committee, "Physical Activity Guidelines Advisory Committee Report, 2008" (Washington, DC: US Department of Health and Human Services, 2008).
5. G.F. Fletcher et al., "Statement on Exercise: Benefits and Recommendations for Physical Activity Programs for all Americans; A Statement for Health Professionals by the Committee on Exercise and Cardiac Rehabilitation of the Council on Clinical Cardiology, American Heart Association," *Circulation* 94 (1996): 857–62.
6. "In Memoriam: Thomas J. Bassler, MD, If You Plan to Remain Sedentary, See Your Doctor First," The Free Library, http://www.thefreelibrary .com/In+memoriam%3A+Thomas +J.+Bassler,+MD+if+you+plan+to +remain+sedentary,...-a0285436344.
7. J. Emmett, "The Physiology of Marathon Running," *Marathon and Beyond*, http://www.marathonand beyond.com/choices/emmett.htm.
8. K. Cooper, *Antioxidant Revolution* (Nashville: Thomas Nelson, 1997).
9. J. Mandrola, "Inflamed Endurance Athletes Should Take No Comfort in Tour De France Cycling Study," *Medscape*, September 3, 2013.
10. J.H. O'Keefe, "Run for Your Life! At a Comfortable Pace, and Not Too Far," TEDxUMKC, November 27, 2012.
11. "Too Much Prolonged High-Intensity Exercise Risks Heart Health," *ScienceDaily*, May 4, 2014, http:// www.sciencedaily.com/releases /2014/05/140514205756.htm.
12. P. Schnohr et al., "Dose of Jogging and Long-Term Mortality: The Copenhagen City Heart Study," *Journal of the American College of Cardiology* 65, no. 5 (2015): 411–19.
13. R.S. Schwartz et al., "Increased Coronary Artery Plaque Volume among Male Marathon Runners," *Missouri Medicine* 111, no. 2 (2014): 85.
14. R.S. Paffenbarger et al., "Physical Activity, All-Cause Mortality, and Longevity of College Alumni," *New England Journal of Medicine* 314, no. 10 (1986): 605–13.

15. K. Helliker, "A Study That Can Help in the Long Run," *Wall Street Journal*, February 12, 2015.

16. G.W. Edson, "Physical Activity and Its Effects on Reducing Disease: A Literature Review of the National Runner's Health Study (2014)," University of Tennessee Honors Thesis Projects, http://trace.tennessee.edu/utk_chanhonoproj/1767. T.M. Eijsvogels et al., "Exercise at the Extremes: The Amount of Exercise to Reduce Cardiovascular Events," *Journal of the American College of Cardiology* 67, no. 3 (2016): 316–29.

CHAPTER 5

1. C.A. Macera, "Lower Extremity Injuries in Runners, Advances in Prediction," *Sports Medicine* 13, no. 1 (1992): 50–57.

2. M.L. Pollock et al., "Effects of Frequency and Duration of Training on Attrition and Incidence of Injury," *Medicine and Science in Sports and Exercise* 9, no. 1 (1977): 31–36.

3. J.M. Hootman et al., "Predictions of Lower Extremity Injury among Recreationally Active Adults," *Clinical Journal of Sport Medicine* 12, no. 2 (2002): 99–106.

4. S.D. Walter et al., "The Ontario Study of Running-Related Injuries," *Archives of Internal Medicine* 149, no. 11 (1989): 2,561–64. C.A. Macera et al., "Predicting Lower-Extremity Injuries among Habitual Runners," *Archives of Internal Medicine* 149, no. 11 (1989): 2,565–68.

5. B. Marti et al., "On the Epidemiology of Running Injuries: The 1984 Bern Grand-Prix Study," *American Journal of Sports Medicine* 16, no. 3 (1988): 285–44.

6. J.E. Taunton et al., "A Prospective Study of Running Injuries: The Vancouver Sun Run 'In Training' Clinics," *British Journal of Sports Medicine* 37, no. 3 (2003): 239–44.

7. M.E. Kasmer et al., "Foot Strike Pattern and Performance in a Marathon," *International Journal of Sports Physiology and Performance* 8, no. 3 (2013): 286–92.

8. A.H. Gruber et al., "Economy and Rate of Carbohydrate Oxidation during Running with Rearfoot and Forefoot Strike Patterns," *Journal of Applied Physiology* 115, no. 2 (2013): 194–201.

9. W.H. Van Mechelen et al., "Is Range of Motion of the Hip and Ankle Joint Related to Running Injuries? A Case Control Study," *International Journal of Sports Medicine* 13, no. 8 (1992): 605–10.

10. T.R. Derrick, J. Hamill, and G.E. Caldwell, "Energy Absorption of Impacts during Running at Various Stride Lengths," *Medicine and Science in Sports and Exercise* 30, no. 1 (1998): 128. J.A. Mercer et al., "Individual Effects of Stride Length and Frequency on Shock Attenuation during Running," *Medicine and Science in Sports and Exercise* 35, no. 2 (2003): 307–13.

11. P.T. Williams, "Effects of Running and Walking on Osteoarthritis and Hip Replacement Risk," *Medicine and Science in Sports and Exercise* 45, no. 7 (2013): 1,292–97.

12. D.E. Hartig and J.M. Henderson, "Increasing Hamstring Flexibility Decreases Lower Extremity Overuse in Military Basic Trainees," *American Journal of Sports Medicine* 27, no. 2 (1999): 173–76.

13. C. Askling, J. Karlsson, and A. Thornstensson, "Hamstring Injury Occurrence in Elite Soccer Players after Preseason Strength Training with Eccentric Overload," *Scandinavian Journal of Medicine and Science in Sports* 13, no. 4 (2003): 244–50.

14. R.W. Willy and I.S. Davis, "The Effect of a Hip-Strengthening Program on Mechanics during Running and during a Single-Leg Squat," *Journal of Orthopaedic and Sports Physical Therapy* 41, no. 9 (2011): 625–32.

15. D.S. Mutton et al., "Effect of Run vs. Combined Cycle/Run Training on VO_2max and Running Performance," *Medicine and Science in Sports and Exercise 1993* 25, no. 12 (1993): 1,393–97. M. Flynn et al., "Cross Training: Indices of Training Stress and Performance," *Medicine and Science in Sports and Exercise* 30, no. 2 (1998): 294–300.

16. R.M. Gabraith and M.E. Lavallee, "Medial Tibial Stress Syndrome: Conservative Treatment Options," *Current Reviews in Musculoskeletal Medicine* 2, no. 3 (2009): 127–33.

17. R. Ferber, K.D. Kendall, and L. Farr, "Changes in Knee Biomechanics after a Hip-Abductor Strengthening Protocol for Runners with Patellofemoral Pain Syndrome," *Journal of Athletic Training* 46, no. 2 (2011): 142–49.

18. E.S. Chumanov et al., "Changes in Muscle Activation Patterns When Running Step Rate Is Increased," *Gait and Posture* 36, no. 2 (2012): 231–35.

19. R.E. Arendse et al., "Reduced Eccentric Loading of the Knee with the Pose Running Method," *Medicine and Science in Sports and Exercise* 36, no. 2 (2004): 272–77.

20. T. Nicholas et al., "Barefoot Running: An Evolution of Current Hypothesis, Future Research, and Clinical Applications," *British Journal of Sports Medicine* 48, no. 5 (2014): 349–55.

21. S.T. Ridge et al., "Foot Bone Marrow Edema after a 10-Week Transition to Minimalist Shoes," *Medicine and Science in Sports and Exercise* 45, no. 7 (2013): 1,363–68.

22. J.J. Knakip et al., "Injury Reduction Effectiveness of Assigning Running Shoes on Plantar Shape in Marine Corps Basic Training," *American Journal of Sports Medicine* 38, no. 9 (2010): 1,759–67.

23. R.M. Nigg et al., "Running Shoes and Running Injuries: Mythbusting and a Proposal for Two New Paradigms: 'Preferred Movement Path' and 'Comfort Filter,'" *British Journal of Sports Medicine 2015* 49, no. 20 (2015): 1,290–94.

24. Marti, "On the Epidemiology of Running Injuries."

CHAPTER 6

1. Noakes, *Lore of Running*.

2. Ibid.

3. Ibid.

4. "Percy Cerutty," Racing Past, http://www.racingpast.ca/john_contents.php?id=93.

5. "Workout Paces and Details," Runbayou, http://www.runbayou.com/ArthurLydiard.pdf.

6. K. Moore, *Bowerman and the Men of Oregon: The Story of Oregon's Legendary Coach and Nike's Cofounder* (New York: Rodale, 2007).

7. J. Daniels, *Daniels' Running Formula* (Champaign, IL: Human Kinetics, 1998).

CHAPTER 7

1. M. Csikszentmihalyi, *Flow: The Psychology of Optimal Experience* (New York: Harper Perennial, 2008).

2. S.R. McClaran, "The Effectiveness of Personal Training on Changing Attitudes Toward Physical Activity," *Journal of Sports Science and Medicine* 2, no. 1 (2003): 10–14.

CHAPTER 8

1. W.J. Pierce and D.E. Pierce, "Who Runs Even Marathon Splits?" *Marathon and Beyond* 7, no. 3 (2003): 66.

2. Noakes, *Lore of Running*.

3. B. Glover and P. Schuder, *The New Competitive Runner's Handbook* (New York: Penguin, 1988).

4. D.L. Costill, *Inside Running: Basics of Sports Physiology* (Canmet, IN: Benchmark Press, 1986).

5. Pierce and Pierce, "Who Runs Even Marathon Splits?"

6. J. Hanc, "Party at My Pace," www.runnersworld.com, September 10, 2008.

7. W.J. Pierce and D.E. Pierce, "Do Marathoners in Pacing Groups Achieve Target Times," *Marathon and Beyond* 7, no. 3 (2003): 84.

CHAPTER 9

1. J.E. Brown, *Nutrition Now* (Belmont, CA: Thomas Wadsworth, 2008), 28: 4.

2. Noakes, *Lore of Running*, 143–63.

3. M. Williams, *Nutrition for Health, Fitness, and Sport* (New York: McGraw-Hill, 2005): 137.

4. Ibid., 138.
5. Ibid.
6. Ibid.
7. Ibid.
8. B. Pierce, S. Murr, and R. Moss, *Runner's World Run Less, Run Faster* (New York: Rodale, 2012): 151.
9. T. Noakes, *Waterlogged: The Serious Problem of Overhydration in Endurance Sports* (Champaign, IL: Human Kinetics, 2012).
10. Williams, *Nutrition for Health, Fitness, and Sport*, 355.
11. Ibid., 356.
12. Ibid.
13. Ibid., 19.
14. Ibid.
15. A. Jeukendrup and M. Gleeson, *Sport Nutrition: An Introduction to Energy Production and Performance* (Champaign, IL: Human Kinetics, 2004): 239.
16. health.gov/dietaryguidelines
17. W.C. Willett, *Eat, Drink, and Be Healthy* (New York: Free Press, 2001).
18. "The Nutrition Source: Healthy Eating Plate and Healthy Eating Pyramid," http://www.hsph.harvard.edu/nutritionsource/healthy-eating-plate/.
19. Ibid.
20. Willett, *Eat, Drink, and Be Healthy*, 179.
21. M. Pollan, *The Omnivore's Dilemma* (New York: Penguin, 2006).
22. Willett, *Eat, Drink, and Be Healthy*, 35.

CHAPTER 10

1. G. Sheehan, *Running and Being: The Total Experience* (New York: Simon and Schuster, 1978): 76.
2. R. Bannister, *The Four-Minute Mile* (Guilford, CT: Lyons Press, 2004): 50.
3. Ibid., 4.
4. Sheehan, *Running and Being*, 72.
5. J. Huizinga, *Homo Ludens: A Study of the Play-Element in Culture* (Boston: Beacon Press, 1938).

6. R. Toor, *Personal Record: A Love Affair with Running* (Lincoln, NB: University of Nebraska Press, 2008).
7. Sheehan, *Running and Being*, 39.
8. S. Mipham, *Running with the Mind of Meditation: Lessons for Training Body and Mind* (New York: Harmony Books, 2012): 148.
9. A. Burfoot, *The Runner's Guide to the Meaning of Life* (New York: Rodale, 2000): 13.
10. Ibid., 57.
11. Mipham, *Running with the Mind of Meditation*, 82.
12. Bannister, *Four-Minute Mile*, 60.
13. Ibid., 201.
14. Mipham, *Running with the Mind of Meditation*, 94.
15. Toor, *Personal Record*, 8.
16. Mipham, *Running with the Mind of Meditation*, 188.

CHAPTER 12

1. R. Nilwik et al., "The Decline in Skeletal Muscle Mass with Aging Is Mainly Attributed to a Reduction in Type II Muscle Fiber Size," *Experimental Gerontology* 48 no. 5, (2013): 492–98.
2. J. Epping et al., *Growing Stronger: Strength Training for Older Adults* (Boston: Tufts University, 2002): 9.

APPENDIX C

Approved by the WMA and USATF

Compiled by Alan Jones with Rex Harvey

AlanLJones@stny.rr.com

http://runscore.com/Alan/AgeGrade.html

APPENDIX D

Approved by the WMA and USATF

Compiled by Alan Jones with Rex Harvey

AlanLJones@stny.rr.com

http://runscore.com/Alan/AgeGrade.html

ABOUT THE AUTHORS

Bill Pierce, Ed.D., LEAD AUTHOR of *Runner's World Run Less, Run Faster* and cofounder of the Furman Institute of Running and Scientific Training (FIRST), is a professor of health sciences at Furman University.

Dr. Pierce, listed as one of 10 marathon "supercoaches" by *Runner's World* magazine, has made hundreds of presentations on fitness, wellness, and running. He and FIRST have been featured in articles in the *Wall Street Journal, New York Times, Business Week, Men's Journal, Runner's World, Hindu,* and many other domestic and international newspapers and magazines.

He joined the Furman University faculty in 1983 and has chaired the department for 32 years. In addition to this administrative role, he has held many leadership positions, including chair of the university faculty.

Dr. Pierce, 67, ran his first of 42 marathons in 1977. He has run the Boston Marathon in five different decades—the 1970s, 1980s, 1990s, 2000s, and 2010s—and through five decades of his life—from his twenties into his sixties. His best time of 2:44 was run at the age of 41.

He graduated from Davidson College in 1971 with a bachelor's degree in political science. He earned a master's degree in sport studies from West Virginia University and a doctorate in health and physical education from Virginia Tech.

Bill's wife, Marianne, is an academic administrator and professor of business administration at Furman.

Scott Murr, Ed.D., is an assistant professor in the health sciences department at Furman University and coauthor of *Runner's World Run Less, Run Faster.* In addition to teaching at Furman, he manages the Molnar Human Performance Lab and is a cofounder of the Furman Institute of Running and Scientific Training (FIRST).

Dr. Murr started running as a teenager when his father joined the running boom in the mid-1970s. Over the past 3 decades, Scott has completed more than 30 marathons and 200 multisport events. He has run a sub-17-minute 5-K, a 2:46 marathon, and a 10:09 Ironman triathlon. He is a 12-time Ironman triathlon finisher (a participant in six World Championships) and has competed on Team USA in the two Duathlon World Championships.

With more than 30 years of experience in the scientific and applied aspects of wellness, fitness, and sports performance, Dr. Murr directs laboratory assessment and designs training programs to help runners succeed.

He graduated from Furman University in 1984 with a bachelor's degree in health and physical education. He earned a master's degree in exercise science from Slippery Rock University in 1993, and a doctorate in exercise science from the University of Georgia in 1997.

Dr. Murr is married to Leslie Fraser, a retired systems analyst. They have two teenage children who keep them quite busy.

INDEX

rest, 138, 140
shoes, 77
strength training, 76, 78
stretching, 76–77
Williams's advice on, xxiii, 71–80, 83
previous, 70, 138
Q&A about, 71–80, 83
runners' attitude about, 70
runners being at risk for, 19–20
"runner's knee," 78
running after recovery from, 82, 98
running fast and, 73
running form and, faulty, 14, 73–74
running surfaces and, 80
shin splints, 77
shoes and, 79
stress fractures, 77–79, 171
stride rate and, 74–75
training and, 70–72
treating, 77–78
Williams's analysis of, 71
Intensity
of exercise, 153–54
of training, xxv–xxvi, 90–91, 150, 152
Interval training, 219–20
Intimacy among runners, 142

J

Joint replacement, 75
Joy of running, xxvi–xxvii, 134–35, 140, 142

K

Knee replacement, 75

L

Lactate threshold, 8–10, 121
Lactate threshold test, 9
Lactic acid accumulation, 109–10
Listening to body, 80, 82
Long-distance running. *See also* Half-marathon; Marathon
Bassler's research on, 57–58, 60
cardiovascular disease and, xxii, 57–58, 61, 63, 66–67
coaching and, 104–5
conclusions about health of, xxii, 66–67
Cooper's research on, 59–60
Emery's recommendations for, 66–67
Fixx and, 60
frequent, 61
health benefits of, 62–65
health debate about, 57–58, 66–67
high-intensity, 61

in interval training, 220
Mandrola's recommendation for, 61
in moderation, 61
O'Keefe's research on, 58, 61
training partner and, 99–100
Longevity and exercise, 63
Lydiard, Arthur, 86

M

Marathon. *See also* Racing; *specific race*
aging and participation in, 29, <u>29</u>
allure of, xxii, 43–44
average time of finishing, 44
as bucket list item, 48
business of, 48–50
charity, 45–47
completing, 48
entry fees, 49
finishing times, median (1980 and 2014), 45
finish-line cutoffs, 44–45
friends and, running with, 50, 52
half-marathon versus, 44
health impact of, 54–55
international, 52–53
joy of, 54
mystery of, xxii, 53
planned pace for, 111–12
scheduling, 137–38
for slow runners, 44–45
split times and, 113–14
travel experience of, 52–53
trend toward running, 43
women runners and, 47–48
Massage, 77
Masters runners, 31, 39–41
Maximal Oxygen consumption (VO$_2$max), 2, 6–8, 14, 32–34
Meal supplement, 124
Medial tibial stress syndrome (MTSS), 77
Meditation, 98
Mileage
injuries and weekly, 72, 87
training, 87–88
Molnar Human Performance Laboratory
assessments at
advantages of, 5–6
body composition, 11–14
gait analysis, 14–16
lactate threshold, 8–10
maximal oxygen consumption, 2, 6–8
overview, 2, 6
performance and, 16–17
training and, 6
FIRST Adult Running and Learning Retreat and, 1–5
McCreesh (John) at, 3–5

R

Racing. *See also* Half-marathon; Marathon; *specific race*
  age-adjusted race time tables and, 37–39, <u>38</u>
  aging and, 27, 29, 39–41
  business of, 48–50
  cancelling participation in, 140
  carbohydrates and, 120
  charity, 45–47
  comparison of current time to world-class time for age and, 251, <u>252–57</u>
  competition of, special, 136–37
  conversion of current time to earlier time equivalent and, 243, <u>244–49</u>
  diet and
    after event, 126
    carbohydrate loading and, 122–23
    day before event, 123–24
    during event, 124–25
    week before event, 122–23
  entry fees, 49
  pace, 107–11
  preparing for, 137–38
  recovery from, 126–27
  road, 49–50
  scheduling, 137–38
  solo running in preparing for, 98
  training and target event for, 88
Range of motion, 152, 191. *See also* Flexibility
Recovery
  cross-training and, 152
  from injury, running after, 82, 98
  from racing, 126–27
  from training, 152
Resistance training. *See* Strength training
Rest in injury prevention, 138, 140
Road races, 49–50. *See also* Racing; *specific race*
Rock 'n' Roll Marathon Series, 49
Rowing workouts
  advantages of, 153
  Monday schedule, 156
  Sunday schedule, 168
  supplemental, 241
  Wednesday schedule, 160
Runners. *See also specific name*; Up Close and Personal
  body weight and, overemphasis on, 172
  Boston Marathon qualifying time as common goal of, 23
  bucket lists of, 48
  finish time goals of, 23, 107, 112
  intimacy among, 142
  Masters, 31, 39–41
  messages sent to FIRST by, xx–xxi
  perceived exertion and, xxvi
  rituals of, 124
  slow, 44–45
  stretching and, 194
  traits of
    achieving goals, 18–19
    being at risk for injuries, 19–20
    being motivated by specific goals, 18
    coaching, benefiting from, 20
    cross-training, failing to be consistent or effective with, 20
    finding identity in running, 17–18
    ignoring potential injuries, 20
    neglecting development of good flexibility, 22
    not training at correct pace, 21–22
    not working on improving form, posture, and gait, 22
    pursuing conflicting goals, 19
    sabotaging efforts with extra body weight, 23
    wanting to qualify for Boston Marathon, 23
  women, 47–48
Runner's knee, 78
Running. *See also* Long-distance running; Run workouts; Solo running; Training
  accountability and, 96
  advantages of, 140–42
  age-adjusted race time tables and, 37–39, <u>38</u>
  aging's impact on
    expectations about, 31–32
    physiological changes, 32–34
    social, cultural, emotional, and mental factors, 34–36
    understanding, xix–xxi
  analysis, 74
  balancing life and, xxvii, 143
  barefoot, 78–79
  boom in, 59–61
  confidence and, 141
  consistency in, 96, 104–5
  days per week of, 90
  discipline and, 130–31, 141
  economy, 14–16, 192
  efficiency, 152
  as egalitarian activity, 69, 137
  fast, xxv, 73, 109, 135–36
  "flow," 98
  friendship and, 141–42
  group, 95–96
  happiness and, 142
  health benefits of, 62–65
  health consequences of not, xxiii
  identity in, finding, 17–18
  injuries as drawback to, xxii, 69
  intimacy among runners and, 142